MAKING SENSE OF MEDICINE

MAKING SENSE OF MEDICINE

Bridging the Gap between Doctor Guidelines and Patient Preferences

Zackary Berger

ROWMAN & LITTLEFIELD
Lanham • Boulder • New York • London

Published by Rowman & Littlefield
A wholly owned subsidiary of The Rowman & Littlefield Publishing Group, Inc.
4501 Forbes Boulevard, Suite 200, Lanham, Maryland 20706
www.rowman.com

Unit A, Whitacre Mews, 26-34 Stannary Street, London SE11 4AB

British Library Cataloguing in Publication Information Available

Library of Congress Cataloging-in-Publication Data

Names: Berger, Zackary, 1973– , author.
Title: Making sense of medicine : bridging the gap between doctor guidelines and patient preferences
    / Zackary Berger.
Description: Lanham : Rowman & Littlefield, [2016] | Includes bibliographical references and index.
Identifiers: LCCN 2015045354 | ISBN 9781442242326 (cloth : alk. paper)
Subjects: | MESH: Patient Participation. | Physician-Patient Relations. | Communication. | Practice
    Guidelines as Topic.
Classification: LCC R727.3 | NLM W 62 | DDC 610.69/6—dc23 LC record available at http://
    lccn.loc.gov/2015045354

∞ ™ The paper used in this publication meets the minimum requirements of
American National Standard for Information Sciences Permanence of Paper for
Printed Library Materials, ANSI/NISO Z39.48-1992.

Printed in the United States of America

To my family, colleagues, friends, teachers, and patients

מײַנע בני־בית, זאָלן זיי לעבן, לאַכן און געזונט זײַן

CONTENTS

INTRODUCTION

Deciding for Yourself

Mrs. T is one of the funniest people I know and also one of the most exasperating. Whenever I run into her, I get a smile on my face—and have to think carefully about what I am going to talk about with her and how, because she is my patient, and the two of us have completely different approaches to life. I am a politically liberal, middle-aged Jew who thinks the Affordable Care Act is great but didn't go far enough. I live in Baltimore City. She lives on the Maryland shore, worries for my safety in the city, and often makes baleful remarks about the government's takeover of health care (from which she benefits). She tells me that she loves Jews, by which she means—I think—that we have a role in the messianic plan of her church.

Recently, I had a conversation with her that was disconcerting and helped motivate the realization that forms the foundation of this book.

Mrs. T had to have surgery on her shoulder. That was an easy case: it had been hurting her for years, and she was very interested in an operation. I referred her to a surgeon. As often happens, the surgeon wanted her to get a number of tests, and among them was an electrocardiogram, a heart tracing. I didn't think she needed it.

She had the shoulder operation without incident.

Afterward, however, her surgeon noticed something that I hadn't on her electrocardiogram—an irregular heart rhythm. I was grateful to him for picking that up, and I had the patient come in to talk about it.

"What's going on with me?" said Mrs. T.

I said, "It looks like you have an irregular heart rate."

"Atrial fibrillation?" she said. "You can use the term with me. My brother has that, and my sister."

We talked about her palpitations and looked through some previous heart tracings. Some of them were normal, and some of them included the irregular rhythm. So we discussed the fact that she likely had paroxysmal atrial fibrillation—that is, an irregular heart rate that is sometimes there and sometimes not.

"What should I do about it?" she asked me.

I said it wasn't clear. She looked at me: What do you mean, it's not clear? "This is your job, Doc," she told me, in her inimitable way. *Let's cut the BS*, she was implying. *I know you are into this sharing the decision making with the patient thing, but surely you know more than I do about such things. You have the technical expertise. So TELL ME WHAT TO DO!*

I said, again, it wasn't clear, and this time she believed me. There are several treatments commonly given to people with atrial fibrillation: anti-coagulation (blood thinner) to help decrease the risk of strokes, medicine to help decrease and regulate the heart rate. She was already on a medication of the second kind to help control her blood pressure. She was more interested in talking about the first category. Again I waffled a bit, wanting to present all of the options to her and not unduly influence her. The problem, however, was that she wanted to be influenced. That is why she was coming to me!

"So," she pressed, "should I be on a blood thinner or not?"

I still wasn't sure. Her rhythm was not continuously irregular, and while the studies, by and large, showed an increased risk of stroke in patients with off-and-on irregular heart rate (paroxysmal atrial fibrillation), as she had, they did not focus on whether treatment with the above medications would have the same risk/benefit balance as for those patients with a continuously irregular heart rate. Again, she got frustrated or impatient with my disinclination to tell her what to do. "Talk with the cardiologist and get back to me."

The cardiologist and I had a very nice chat, convincing me that blood thinners were a reasonable decision in this patient and that I shouldn't be so reluctant to use them. But it turned out, when talking to Mrs. T later, that she was in fact a little worried about the risks of bleeding (she

enjoyed playing squash and worried that she might run up against something and bleed spontaneously). She knew that the newer blood thinners
were more difficult to reverse with antidotes, as opposed to the tried-and-
true warfarin (brand name Coumadin) used by many people, albeit requir-
ing regular blood checks.

She decided, in the end, that she would look things up and get back to
me. Between the time of our chat and the time we next talked, she did
look up some facts about anticoagulation and their risks and benefits.
More important, she spoke to her relatives: she has a sister whose husband was diagnosed with atrial fibrillation and tried warfarin for a while
but decided to discontinue it because of what he had read about bleeding.

She called me back the next week with two decisions: one, she did not
want to start any blood thinner right now, and two, she wanted to avoid
the new anticoagulations that her cardiologist had recommended.

All of the information in the world did not move her to make one
decision or the other until she talked to her family members and heard
their stories. The data did not move her—narrative did. It is still not clear
to me, even after all of the talk that doctors and patients should be equal
partners in treatment decisions, who in fact made the decision here: me,
her, or her cardiologist. Was it the cardiologist, who recommended that
she take a blood thinner? Was it me, who discussed the cardiologist's
recommendations with her and added my reservations? Or was it her,
who was either delaying or actually researching her options?

What should she do?

In the context of health care, this has been presented in the past few
decades as an instance either of decision making, on the one hand, or, on
the other hand, of evidence-based medicine.

Shared decision making, as both a concept and a movement, provides
important criteria to make sure that Mrs. T is well supported in this
situation. We should be provided with reliable, unbiased information
communicated in a way we can understand, whereupon we can—if we
are empowered enough and have the right resources—make a decision
that is right for us. The aspects of decision making that are relevant to
health care are many: there are often options to choose among; information does matter; we feel like we have to do something in the right way
for the right reasons; and there is—as for many other important mo-
ments—a feeling of fate and associated trauma. We need to have some-

one there to make the decision with us so that we are not abandoned but so that—at the same time—our autonomy is acknowledged and sustained.

Another approach to the problems of health care is that of evidence-based medicine (EBM). The best science should be used to drive our health care. We want the best studies, using the most reliable scientific methods, to find what works for us.

The big secret of health care, which this book is meant to unpack, is that neither of these rubrics work completely. They both miss big parts of what it's like to be sick or to be a person trying to preserve one's own health.

Decision making is important, but it is not the whole story; not everything that we seek when getting care has to do with decision making. We look for care, a sense that our desires and preferences are being taken into account, and a guide. We want presence on the journey as much as we want a particular destination. No matter how deeply I have drunk from the well of shared decision making and try to converse with patients on that basis, there are still many who want me to give them a recommendation. This might be because they are not used to the concept that they can make their own decisions—that is, either they do not feel empowered enough or I have not given them the power to participate—or just because people need and want guidance.

In the first decades of the EBM movement, the motivation was clear: to remove physician lore, encrusted practices without any basis or merely on the basis of physician say-so, and to add back those practices that were known to work—to use the best achievements of science to treat us on an empirical basis.

If you ask Mrs. T, she will tell you that she does not have much inclination to study the medical literature. Even when I gave her options regarding her treatment, she tended to tell me that it was my responsibility to guide her through the forbidding thickets of scientific literature. "It's on you, Doc," she said, in her inimitable way.

Then we, as patients, have a dilemma. We would like our doctors' thought processes to be transparent so that we know they are helping us make the right decision. But the so-called scientific literature is full of holes, as we will examine in the chapters that follow, for a number of common medical conditions.

Thus, either rubric—shared decision making or evidence-based medicine—is not enough to cover all of our individual health care needs. What we want, and need, is personal care, making us feel better (cared for) in the context of a relationship that enables us to act according to our preferences.

Personal care does not mean tailoring every possible treatment to our genes or protein makeup (which is impossible), nor does it mean abandoning us to a menu of options that we do not fully understand. It means figuring out what our priorities are—but, more important (and perhaps more complicated), also figuring out the structure of our lives and how we can best navigate our health needs given those constraints.

This has several implications regarding our relationships with our doctors and how we approach our health conditions. To figure out how this might work, let's talk to Ms. B, who works at an international airport, has a three-year-old daughter, and has been married for ten years.

She was diagnosed with diabetes recently and thought that she was destined to a life of insulin, a prospect that terrified her (many people can get used to insulin, but it turned out not to be right for her). But the circumstances of her life made it possible, and necessary, to reexamine her assumptions.

She came, first of all, to tell me that she had been diagnosed with diabetes with another doctor a year before (I had not been aware of the diagnosis). Her life was falling apart, she said, and she didn't know how she could manage to be on a therapy that required her to inject herself every day.

She also wasn't ready to check her sugars every day, she said, and she was not sure she knew how to treat her diabetes at all.

It turns out that she was depressed and had been for a long time, but she wasn't sure whether any of the treatment options we discussed might work for her.

At this moment, with her diabetes and depression (which are known to interact and lead to worse outcomes than either alone),[1] are we speaking about some sort of decision to be made, whether to treat her diabetes or depression? Surely not—Ms. B would like them to get better. The question is not whether she would like to deal with them but how she is to live with them.

Are we asking what the best evidence tells us about treating someone like Ms. B? In this case, we should ask what "best evidence" means. For many doctors and researchers, best evidence is derived from a scientific trial of a certain sort, in which two groups of patients are randomized to two different treatments so that, on average, the characteristics of the two groups won't vary, leaving the treatment the only thing that differs between them and thus making it possible for the scientist or statistician to isolate the effect of the first treatment compared to the second.

There are no trials of Ms. B's case, however, for the simple reason that Ms. B is unique. There are studies of the best treatments of diabetes and the best treatments of depression, but there are no randomized controlled trials, that I am aware of, for the best treatments for people who have both diabetes and depression. Thus, there is no best answer to the question, What is the best route to take: to treat diabetes first, so as to have fewer clinical symptoms of high blood sugar, or to treat depression first?

Evidence-based medicine is often over *there*, in a space where rigorous trials are conducted with the help of committed patients. In the real world, studies about complicated people and multiple problems are often not to be found, and the balance of risks and benefits is very different.

The other dogma, shared decision making, takes us in the other direction, assuming empowered people who are engaged in every detail and *want* such engagement. We know that not everyone is this way—Mrs. T wanted explicit direction toward a decision.

This book talks about what to do in the space between. If we are unique individuals, it does not follow that we are to be sluiced down the pipe of so-called shared decision making when we neither have nor are interested in the details of treatments and side effects, about which doctors might think they are supposed to educate us before making a decision on our behalf.

If we are people living in a science-centric society, where we expect doctors to use the latest information on our behalf (itself an assumption and ideology worth questioning), it does not follow that our concerns should be shoehorned into the rubric of evidence-based medicine.

This book is about how to find that space in between and navigate it for the benefit of our own interests and of those around us. It is also about how to keep our identity as people when our diseases tend to depersonalize us. It is about how to help the most disadvantaged find that space as well, for the benefit of all of us.

How do we navigate? Not through absenting ourselves from the system—because there is no live alternative that will provide better care for individuals and communities—and not through adversarially demanding "better care," but by understanding the uncertainties associated with medicine and using this understanding to our advantage.

If you, by definition, are not average (since you are an individual), then you have particular needs and preferences, which you must take into account when choosing your health care. This book will tell you how to do this in the context of individual common diseases. But there is more. Our individual responsibilities do not stop at our own health records, medicines, health outcomes, and prescriptions. We are also responsible for the health of those around us because their health affects ours and the opportunities available to us.

The more people I see in my function as a general internist and primary care doctor, the more I realize that individual health and public health are not as easily distinguishable as might be assumed by our larger institutions and government agencies. That is, each of us can be responsible in a positive sense for the health of those around us.

You will see the outlines of such an approach in the following chapters:

1. *Pay attention to the consequences of health care decisions on resources.*

   Ms. D is a fifty-four-year-old woman with chronic back pain who has had no fewer than six MRIs. She did not realize that an MRI is an advanced imaging technology and that the number of MRIs done for lower back pain runs to millions of dollars per year.

2. *Realize that health care inequities are based on a history of institutional racism, which can affect how we view care.*

   Does this affect your care? If you are a member of a minority or disadvantaged group, it would be lovely to think that our society and health care disparities will improve themselves to a degree that will be noticeable in your lifetime. Failing that—and far be it for me, as a privileged white doctor, to direct your care—it might behoove you to seek ways in which you can help address the gaps in care due to disparities. If you are white, is your care affected by disparities? Absolutely. Health care disparities have to do with an entire culture of inequities and are founded on the notion that some groups of people are worth more than others. And, by the same token, our system assumes that "a certain amount" of care is better than a lesser amount. More or more prestigious care is held to be better, and those who get less of it are held to be worse off. Thus, we are told that we should take advantage of that "more."

If we recognized the powerful forces of inequality that have dictated the structure of our health care system, we might realize that more is not better and that placing everyone on an equal footing of communication and empathy would lead to equivalent or even improved outcomes and that the very outcomes themselves should be built around what each person needs.

If Ms. D knew that "best care" for her back pain does not necessarily include an MRI, perhaps her expectations would be different and she would be better prepared to deal with the reality of an on-again, off-again, chronic, though non-life-threatening, illness, without thinking that there is some "higher level of care" out there.

3. *Do not expect too much from medical science.*

The greatest successes of medical science in the twentieth century were significant indeed: the elimination of diseases such as smallpox and, though not yet complete, polio; reducing the risk of death from heart disease; and the list goes on. Mortality from infectious diseases has also been decreased.

But the weaknesses of medical science are also obvious: the troubling ethical lapses associated with unethical experimentation on human beings; the massive investments in and promotion of interventions that do not bear much clinical relevance or aid to the health of the population (cf. the Human Genome Project and similar claims made today about precision medicine).

Without addressing the too-broad question about comparing the risks and benefits of medical science, any claim about the linear progress of medical science is complicated at best. The fact that many of us cannot get the care we need or know of ways in which we were treated unfairly—not given good care by our doctor or unable to reach care by a doctor, not given useful medicine, subjected to tests that, in the short or long run, did not seem to help at all—tells us that medical science does not help as much as it is supposed to, and it is certainly not any panacea for our individual or community health.

We will thus revisit the assumption that medical science progresses ever forward and try to see what the imperfection of biomedical science and its intermittent inability to provide useful answers has to do with our personal strategies to deal with and hopefully improve our health conditions.

In short, much that health care professionals do to and for us is unproven by rigorous science—and the portion that is might not apply to us in particular. Many conditions that we encounter in our daily life, if they are not dangerous or acute, are things that either might get better on their own or are not susceptible to the types of advanced treatments that many doctors may offer to us.

We live in a culture of multiple possible tests and treatments, many of which are available even if they have not been proven to work. We have inflated expectations about the value of science, and we are dubious of any potential treatment that does not bear its imprimatur.

Mrs. T still has not been back in touch with me with her decision about whether to be on a blood thinner. I called her back once, but she has not returned the call. I think that is okay. She is deciding in a way that is right for her—and that means not making a decision right now. Whether or not she has really internalized the potential risk of stroke, she has definitely "voted with her feet" about the potential harms of blood thinner—that is, bleeding.

Deciding for yourself is what this book is all about.

I

CHRONIC PAIN

Many Treatments, No Solution

Understanding what it is like to be sick means starting with the story of someone who is sick. Every person is different. When a system is set up to bring the best health to populations, even the best of intentions may not ensure that care is tailored to the individual. How do we bridge what a doctor knows to be true, on the basis of science, and what a patient is convinced is the case from their own experience? We will start with one story that introduces us to a whole volume of such conflicts—fruitful episodes of cognitive dissonance in the health care setting. Understanding these stories might nudge us closer to an understanding of care that respects the individual while still taking advantage of scientific advances derived from population science.

Let's take pain. A system that assumes that everyone with pain has the same needs or weaknesses is likely to find drug addiction where none exists or to give out medication where none is needed. Mr. Wheeler is sixty-five years old and has a list of diseases that stretches down the page, from diabetes to gout, depression to congestive heart failure. He has not held a job in about nine months, and his relationship with his wife is under stress. She lost her job, too, for reasons that have nothing to do with Mr. Wheeler's medical condition. They are about to lose their home. He frequently mentions his eleven-year-old son, and his love and pride for the boy are evident.

Mr. Wheeler is not working because of his pain. He has chronic nerve-related pain in his right leg, which causes swelling and discomfort. For weeks at a time, he is unable to walk on the leg, and he accurately, even a little coldly, describes the shooting pains that render him immobile. Whenever he comes in to see me, we dwell on the leg for nearly the entire length of the visit, leaving aside the many chronic conditions that we should discuss.

Mr. Wheeler and I always have a nice chat when he comes to see me. His wife is pleasant, ready with a smile and a good word about the high level of care that she knows we at Johns Hopkins provide. Sometimes I wonder if she is doing so prophylactically, to make sure that her husband's doctor measures up to the standards for which our institution should stand. Her husband has been out of work for a comparatively short time. There is considerable pressure on him, perhaps from her (though I am not privy to the internal couple dynamic). But his wife usually smooths the path to what turns out to be the subject of discussion at many a visit: what we can do about his leg.

At the same time that I attempt to offer comfort and a sense of healing, working with the patient assiduously to try and minimize his symptoms, we must both realize—at different paces—that there is no cure. Indeed, thinking that there is a cure might lead to problems even worse than the disease. However, refusing to offer some amelioration, or hope, is a betrayal of the trust that Mr. Wheeler has placed in me.

Despite the chronic, ongoing nature of this gentleman's pain and its refusal to recede before an ever-shifting array of partial treatments over many years, it would be a mistake to surrender to any personal nihilistic tendencies of mine, suggesting that I can do nothing to help this man. He is on a number of medications: metoprolol to help his blood pressure; Xanax to treat his anxiety; Flonase, a steroid, to improve his runny nose, which irritates his throat and causes problems sleeping. He also takes nortriptyline, a kind of antidepression medication. While the pharmaceutical industry rightly gets a bad name, it does produce medications that help.

Even though each of the medications I just listed has its downsides and complications, Mr. Wheeler perceives them as offering him significant aid. He knows that his depression has improved since starting the nortriptyline; he can get through an anxiety attack since starting the Xanax. We talk together about his blood pressure frequently, and we both agree it is now better controlled—even with the caveat that someone with his level of blood pressure, on the basis of the available evidence, may or may not be clearly helped by medication, in the sense of benefiting from reduced risk of stroke or heart attack.

By the same token, he is on a number of medicines to treat his pain, and they have helped him significantly. His gabapentin has reduced his nerve pain, although it has not resolved it completely. He is on a Lidoderm patch, which also takes the edge off somewhat.

When he first met me, he came to me with a number of prescriptions that had been started by other doctors. Two of them were oxycodone and morphine. His morphine was long-acting—he only had to take one pill a day. His oxycodone was short-acting—he took one pill every few hours. These were pills for chronic pain.

When I saw these pills on his medication list, my heart sank. I knew what the findings of evidence-based medicine showed: opiates (a type of medication that includes oxycodone and morphine) are not effective in chronic pain, or at least no more effective than anti-inflammatory medicines (NSAIDS).[1]

I knew this because the literature—scholarly, directed at the lay public, and educational materials aimed at health care providers—told me at length about the dangerous opiate epidemic that was currently, like the rising sea levels that are the product of global warming, lapping at the shores of America's sick, dependent, and poor, sucking them below the surface. Pharmaceutical companies were encouraging doctors to prescribe these medications, and patients dependent on them were helping doctors overlook their misgivings and refill the prescriptions over and over again.[2]

So I reacted predictably—with sympathy and a listening ear but no little certainty. Then, however, I learned later, from the very same scholarly literature, that a different balance obtains in the treatment of nerve-related pain. In fact, there is some evidence that opiates can help in such pain over the short term.[3]

Thus, looking back at the first visit with Mr. Wheeler, I had spent at least a few minutes in my most didactic, non-patient-centric mode, telling him why opiates wouldn't work at all. Then, by the next visit, I had found out that for some patients with nerve-related pain, opiates can work—at least in the short term. The evidence was incomplete, and I was veering to and fro. Mr. Wheeler took this all in stride, believing in me because I was his doctor and knew better.

Then came another look at the evidence—the same review of the literature, which I had not read thoroughly the first time—before the next visit: in the long term, the effectiveness of opiates was subject to "unavoidable uncertainty." So, in essence, we were back to the same place. Thanks either to a previous positive experience he had had with another physician or to his perception that these pain medications had helped him deal with a chronic condition, Mr. Wheeler was not about to give up or reduce the dose of his opiates—at least not on this visit.

At the same time, as a physician who felt bound to follow the dictates of evidence-based medicine, I found myself unable to completely agree with his preferences. Thus, I was caught between two broadly accepted orthodoxies of my profession, and I had no idea what to do. Nor did common practice help me out with some obvious answer or clear advice. What I decided, in the end, did not make me feel perfectly confident in either dogma.

What did I end up doing? Before I get into that question, I want to go back to address the conflict at the core of present-day medicine between evidence and preference, decisions and care, and how that might apply to the treatment of pain.

Pain is more complicated than it first appears. We do not know why one person's pain threshold is lower or higher than another's, nor do we know the precise pathways that explain how damage or stimuli encountered by peripheral nerves can alter pain perceptions in the central nervous system. Of course, there is considerable research into the neurobiology of pain and, especially these days, functional imaging that can trace the changes in brain metabolism during an episode of pain.[4]

But in a larger sense, the treatment of pain is a specific instance of the situation we encounter for many common health problems. Occasionally there are breakthroughs, but the overall picture remains the same. Mr. Wheeler will always suffer from his pain, and while I can vary the particular menu of options available to him, I will never be able to assure him that we will make his pain go away entirely.

If I were to choose a treatment that works well for the broadest cross-section of patients with chronic pain, it would be the treatment that many chronic-pain practitioners have proposed multiple times in the scientific literature: treatment centered on the patient setting individual goals for himself or herself, avoiding medications that encourage dependence, optimizing the patient's mental health, and staying physically active. Such multidisciplinary regimens, including cognitive behavioral therapy, have been extensively reviewed.[5]

Why isn't such a course of treatment a realistic option for this patient? Why do so many patients have recourse to opioids? More important, why do doctors disdain these medications at the same time that many patients see them as their only cure?

The questions and answers for the case of chronic pain are similar to those for other common conditions, laying out the contours for the complications and contradictions that are found at every turn of our modern health care delivery.

PAIN TREATMENT TODAY AND HOW WE GOT HERE

I will not indulge here in a comprehensive history of pain, which this book is too limited to encompass. A number of excellent, recent books cover this story in detail from a theoretical, historical, and patient-narrative perspective. What is more important to recount now is how we got here and how people with chronic pain live their lives.

Like the other common conditions we will discuss in this book, chronic pain is a long-lasting condition, often lifelong, which in the worldview of contemporary medicine is understood as a disease to be cured, not a condition to be sympathized with and healed.[6]

A condition to be cured—as chronic pain is still viewed by many doctors—requires a definitive diagnosis. There must be a reason, because a particular derangement of the organism (to use Thomas Sydenham's terminology[7]) requires a solution particular to that cause. However, in many cases of chronic pain, there is no single discoverable cause.[8]

Many patients have come to me with, for example, chronic back pain, asking through their clear discomfort and frustration "what is going on?"—that is, what is the cause of their back pain. On the one hand, of course, it is a natural thing to desire a full account of what is causing our suffering. Knowing a diagnosis is therapeutic, though I do not know whether this therapeutic information works because the patient thus knows that someone cares about their suffering or because he or she desires a specific reason.

But such searching for causes—especially in certain common conditions that we will explore here—can be counterproductive. It can lead to an ever-widening spiral of tests, which can reinforce this constant causal reaching. It can lead to frustration when a cause is not found. And it can cause recourse to specialists, who are often yoked to this causal search. Most important, such a search can lead away from the search for symptomatic improvement.

There are many methods available today to treat chronic pain and identify potential causes. The number of "pain centers" in the United States has increased over past years; though recent, reliable figures are difficult to come by, they numbered in the hundreds in the 1990s and continue to increase.[9] Most assuredly, they lead the customer-patient to believe that their pain will be improved. But underlying their efforts is the customary medical emphasis on diagnosis and treatment of a single, defined condition.

There are, of course, scientific advances being made in the field of pain control and pain research. There are specialties and exciting lab work. I am not an expert in these fields. However, as a generalist physician, I do know about the day-to-day treatment of patients with chronic pain. The biggest elephant in the room is always opioids, a class of medication that provides great benefit and causes great harm. Unfortunately, neither advocates of the medication nor its passionate detractors can lead us to a one-size-fits-all solution for the treatment of pain.

OPIOIDS

What They Are and Why They Help

The evidence shows that opioids (also called opiates and narcotics) are not more effective than anti-inflammatory medications for the treatment of chronic pain.[10] Yet they are used routinely for acute, painful conditions and are a boon to those suffering from terminal illnesses like cancer.[11]

However, the line between acute and chronic pain is not as sharp as one might think. If a person has many episodes of pain, clearly delineated one from the other, but those episodes never stop, is that pain acute or chronic? On the other hand, if someone has pain that never goes away but only sometimes makes it impossible for that person to feel like they have a normal daily life, is that pain chronic or acute?[12]

Patients routinely tell me that opiates are the only drugs that work for them—there is nothing else that even touches their pain. They tell stories of trudging through medication after medication that does not help, and then—often through a relative's shared prescription, an emergency room visit, or a surgical procedure—they suddenly found opiates. Many know the theoretical considerations that militate against chronic use of such medication but still choose to take it.

It is a strict, ideological mind that can see these people and be determined to discontinue as many of these medications as possible.

Yet Opiates Have Serious Problems

If it is undisputed that opiates can bring powerful benefits, it is almost as undisputed that their chronic use has led to massive problems, such as a steadily advancing wave of misuse and addiction.[13] This has caused death, disease, and strain on both human beings and the system that is supposed to care for them.[14]

The figures have been publicized widely. The yearly number of opiate deaths is greater than the number of deaths from motor vehicle accidents.[15] There are millions of new opiate prescriptions yearly because doctors are prescribing these medications much more frequently than they were before. However, this is not because the medical evidence has crowned them with effectiveness in treating chronic pain.

How Do We Bridge the Two?

It is not easy, either as a person seeing doctors or as a doctor (or other health care provider), to get from the best medical evidence to the person in the room waiting to be helped. There are plenty of public policy solutions for the problem of overprescription of opiates and no shortage of providers, organizations, and researchers proposing them. However, in the moment of the visit, they all disappear in front of the person who is in pain.

Recognizing individual suffering is a basic part of medicine. Bridging the contradiction between evidence-based medicine (what the science says) and patient-centered care (what ordinary people want) is not often discussed in medical schools or training programs. Yet we must do more than register the contradictions; we have to discuss how to bridge this gap.

Understanding the commonalities that link common conditions, as well as the contradictions between evidence, preference, and the care of individuals, may help us make sense of each of these conditions in particular.

BETWEEN EVIDENCE-BASED MEDICINE AND PATIENT-CENTERED CARE

Let me explain what I mean about the contradictions involved in taking care of someone like Mr. Wheeler and, additionally, the difficulties involved in living with a common condition.

Mr. Wheeler is in pain every day. Some days are worse, and some are better. Depending on how you count medications, he has been on half a dozen or more just to treat his pain and jumped from one to the other and back again. He says (and this is a real quote from one of my patients) that he "feels like [he] will always live with it; it is always there."

There are the medications, the constant presence of the pain, its worsening and improvement—sometimes for unclear reasons. There is the chore of changing the medication in the hopes that some edge can be gained on the pain. There are, of course, the regular discussions with his physician—me—about the downsides of using opiates chronically, when I marshal the reasons, which I will discuss below, why they don't help and even hurt in the long run.

But since Mr. Wheeler is reasonably sure that these medications are the only thing that work for him, in the best case these conversations are genteel assurances for myself, his doctor, that a modicum of professional standards are employed. In the worst case, these conversations become awkward exercises in unsaid assumptions, fears, and frustrations. On the one hand, there are my (his physician's) worries about the habit-forming nature of opiates. Even if we agreed to taper him off these medications—that is, decrease them little by little until we were able to discontinue them entirely—we might not be able to make this work practically because of his dependence and the disruption that withdrawal from opiates might cause. (While withdrawal from opiates is generally not as severe as that from other substances, it still can be disruptive.) On the other hand, there are Mr. Wheeler's fears that he might be seen as an addict and his frustration with not being able to stop taking medicines for his chronic pain.

This is my description, based on my time with Mr. Wheeler and patients like him, of the way in which he recounts his experience. But there is a difference between my understandings of his experience, his own narrative of his experience, and, finally, his experience itself, what it is like to be a person with this condition. This last item is something that we need to piece together from a variety of sources: the patient's narrative, the empiric evidence of the scientific literature, and the empathy built in us by nonscientific and more humane and qualitative ways of understanding a fellow human being's experiences.

None of these alone is enough. Health care providers can no longer talk only to each other. By the same token, though, patients' voices, though obviously essential, are not the only ones that matter. Care is a partnership. Thus, we have to assemble evidence of many kinds in order to understand how to relate the story of a patient to the best care available by medicine. This is subjective, just like any narrative.

This subjectivity can make the meeting of an individual and the health care system insurmountably difficult. On the one hand, we have the population-based studies of opiate misuse and the resulting deaths and disease. We have the trials comparing various kinds of pain treatments. But we have nothing that can help us bridge the gap between the subjective experience of a given individual and the scientific evidence, itself often limited, with which the doctor or nurse is confronted.

Let me trace the steps by which a health care provider—a doctor, nurse, or anyone else who might see a patient on a regular basis for a chronic complaint—might approach the treatment of a patient's pain. (The category of health care provider, of course, includes physician assistants and advanced practice nurses; for example, nurse practitioners.)

The first step is to listen to the person with the pain. Then the algorithm can take at least two different turns. The doctor and patient might (ideally, together) decide that the pain is something that should be addressed according to the biomedical model.[16]

According to this model, every derangement of the human organism can be classified as a disease—and diseases, by their nature, are imbalances that should be fixed. We can only fix a disease if we know the cause. So, in the treatment of pain, applying the biomedical model would mean finding out what sort of pain it is through an exact discussion with the patient of the symptoms' characteristics: where it is located, what the nature of the pain is, what brings it on, what makes it worse, where (and whether) it radiates to a certain location, and, finally, what improves it.

The model continues with the physical exam, a procedure hallowed by ritual. The exam is essential to the doctor-patient relationship and to the patient's feelings that he or she is being healed. It can also help determine the cause of pain, especially of acute pain. The underuse of the physical exam is well known and has become a cause célèbre for some.[17]

Next, for many patients with chronic pain, a multitude of tests are conducted in order to get to the bottom of the pain and uncover the fundamental cause, which will hopefully lead in turn to fundamental treatment and a real symptomatic improvement for the patient. These can include imaging (for example, CT scans or MRIs), tests of nerve and muscle function, and functional tests—that is, tests that are meant to evaluate how well the system in question, the one that is producing the pain and other symptoms, actually works.

According to this approach, the tests will lead us to identify the system that is malfunctioning, and then the practitioner can step in and provide an intervention that can fix things. Some abnormal results are usually found. The abnormality may be deceptive, a reflection of statistical laws that any test can produce a "false positive."

There is also another possibility: The testing does find malfunction in a certain system; this result is real (i.e., it is not a false positive), but it is not relevant to the patient's chronic pain. Worse still, in some circumstances, the test result is potentially, marginally, arguably relevant. It is easy to think it might be relevant. It is a promise of a body system that can be fixed to improve the pain.

This arguable relevance provides an inviting signpost to follow. Let's say you are a woman in your fifties with chronic pain in your abdomen, worse with food. Like millions of others, you have been told that this pain might be due to acid reflux. And you have been prescribed the medications known as proton pump inhibitors, which are of partial effectiveness for reflux (resolving symptoms in four weeks in one-third of patients who do not have ulcers[18]). However, your pain still has not resolved completely, although on a good day you could say that it has considerably improved.

Your doctor recommends that you get an image of your abdomen, just in case. Indeed, the CT scan finds something. You have gallbladder stones. What is the relationship between these stones and your chronic abdominal pain? There are probabilities, of course: studies of people like you, clarifying the frequency of gallstones among them. There are even some studies, though few, asking how many of those people with stones experienced improved symptoms after their gallbladder was removed (there is effectiveness in about half of patients [19]).

Unfortunately, there is nothing that can definitively answer the question that you and your doctor really want answered: What is the intervention that will make your pain go away? And if you can accept the answer—probably nothing will make it go away, or at least nothing for sure—then what is the answer to the follow-up: What will make your pain as bearable as possible for the lifetime for which this condition, this kind of life, is going to last?

There are different kinds of answers to this question and different kinds of wisdom that medical science can bring to bear. In this book, we will also talk about the experiences of people who live with these diseases and what their experiences can teach us about living with a common illness.

2

COMMON CONDITIONS

The Gap between Knowledge and Preference

When medications appear that seem to be effective in treating a condition as prevalent and disruptive as pain, both providers and patients start using them without attention to long-term consequences. In recent decades, opiates have become an ever more common treatment for chronic pain, though discomfort over their use is widespread.[1]

This sequence of events is not unique to chronic pain but follows a pattern shared by many common conditions. We can tell a similar story about care for patients at the end of life: technology makes possible choices that did not exist before and that both patients and providers are unprepared to address. One way to address this disconnect between what we can do technologically and what we know how to do emotionally is to educate patients and providers toward a culture change in which patients better recognize the risks and benefits of each option and how those options relate to their preferences.

Culture change is hard. When we are a person with one of these common conditions, or a person tasked to take care of such a patient, how do we live with this gap between knowledge and preference, between technology and decision making, in the moment before our society has achieved the necessary culture change to communicate risks and benefits in the context of individual preferences?

WHAT ARE CHRONIC CONDITIONS?
SOME DEFINITIONS AND COMPLICATIONS

The common conditions we will discuss in this book are customarily called *chronic diseases*. However, this term is inexact. There are diseases that flare up all of a sudden, run their course, and are never heard from again (e.g., urinary tract infections or pneumonia), but, by the same token, these very same diseases can, in sicker people, happen time and again with greater severity and frequency and sometimes cannot be cured with the same effectiveness as in healthier people.

There are other diseases that can lie dormant in the body for years, never becoming evident physically or symptomatically—for example, prostate cancer. Other conditions can be present for a lifetime, making themselves felt in flares or attacks but not noticeable at other times. Then, further, there are diseases like diabetes, which, if cancer is the "emperor of maladies," is the mogul of sickness: doling out complications like a gang lord to different parts of the body.

The binary misnomer of acute versus chronic ailments overshadows the actual experience of illness as lived by the person. If your pain is chronic, it becomes open to dismissal, something about which not much can be done, a burden that must be lived with—a synonym of the dreaded "multiple medical problems" with which many a person is labeled by doctors. The incompleteness of this dichotomy is emphasized by the fact that the medical profession only uses the word *chronic* to modify certain conditions: there is no such thing as "chronic diabetes," for example (at least not in doctors' language), nor "chronic heart failure" or "chronic hypertension."

Chronic is a term used for conditions that are considered outside the realm of the customary paradigm of the biomedical model: diseases are diagnosed, and then they are susceptible to cure.

What happens when diseases last one's whole life, do not introduce themselves as clearly "acute" or "chronic," and do not make it conveniently clear in advance how they are going to change the lives of those who must bear them? What happens for the health care practitioner who takes care of someone with a disease like this, who often must navigate a space that does not exist in the journals of evidence-based medicine and the neat columns of guideline tables? This book is about that space, and this chapter will introduce us to the spectrum of diseases that are to be found there.

Diseases for Which There Is No Cure

This is possibly the largest, most frustrating, and perhaps the most over-looked category of disease. Many definitions of *cure* have been advanced, whether it be addressing the symptoms, uprooting the underlying cause of disease at the organ or system level, or replacing the defect in the molecule or gene that is at fault. However, as we expand and deepen our diagnostic abilities and the resources devoted to them, we realize that more and more of the diseases we find are not susceptible to cure. Hypertension can be due to secondary causes, and if those causes are treated, the hypertension may be resolved. But primary hypertension, once diagnosed, is not generally something that resolves: customarily, a patient is counseled that he or she must take medications for the balance of his or her life.[2] Similarly, although migraine headaches can be resolved,[3] the treatments offered are only with difficulty called a "cure" since they involve the long-term and often daily use of medications.

There are diseases that represent not the dysfunction of a system (like hypertension) or an unsupportable symptom (like migraines), but rather a natural physiological development that is almost impossible to avoid. Osteoarthritis results from degeneration of the cartilage and the underlying bone, which becomes more common with age. Certain factors that make a person more likely to develop arthritis, including obesity/over-weight, leg-length inequalities, malalignment, and trauma, are difficult to avoid or control, as anyone who has had any of these factors can attest.

Labeling a disease *incurable* can mean various things, revealing the weakness of relying too much on the designation *curable*. An incurable cancer is frequently a synonym for a terminal condition. But in the sense above, many conditions that are seen over the course of a lifetime by a primary care provider are ones to which the concept of *cure* does not clearly apply.

How do we approach such conditions, which might be present for years at a time? How do we acknowledge their presence, sometimes unfelt but always realized, in our own life or the life of someone we care for? How do we treat them in a way that recognizes both the person's preferences and the imperfect medical evidence? All these are questions we will discuss, if not definitively answer.

Diseases for Which There Might Be a Cure, But It Is Unclear, Impossible to Know in Advance, and Uncertain Whether That Cure Might Actually Help

Then there are those situations in which some sort of intervention can be offered, but it's not clear whether it will help. To return to the case of back pain: I used to think it was simply a bad idea to have recourse to advanced radiologic imaging (e.g., CTs or MRIs) in the case of garden-variety back pain without red flags. My colleagues and I even published a paper about it.[4] And in most cases, I am still of that opinion.

But I have adopted the same logic, in some cases, that many patients and providers are convinced by. With a few years of practice, and a modicum more of modesty, I have dropped some of the ideological clothing and realized that perhaps some patients are helped by surgical spinal interventions.

I am not going back on the proposition of our article or the efforts of the Less Is More movement. The prevalence of such procedures is completely out of keeping with the evidence present for them on the basis of properly conducted randomized trials. I have come to realize, though, that for individual patients there is always a "however." There is always, somewhere in a big mass of people, that individual for whom an invasive intervention—expensive, involved, and often a failure—actually does work.

Unfortunately, oftentimes our system promotes wholesale interventions as if they will work for many or even most people when they are truly aimed at an unknowable number of individuals—that is, treatments are only partially effective in trials, and then, in the transition from trials to real life, their effectiveness is further reduced.

Cancer provides an example. For a given patient, it is often well-nigh impossible to predict in advance and with perfect certainty whether a given regimen will achieve a cure. Thus, cancer treatments often fall into this category, when it is "unclear, impossible to know in advance, and uncertain whether that cure might actually help."

On the basis of the above discussion, we come to realize that a cure is not necessarily the right goal for everyone. By the same token, diagnosis might not be the right goal for everyone, either. Perhaps the goal is to know enough to feel secure in the problem, or to be told what symptomatic relief might mean, or to understand how family history or mode of life might have contributed to the problem. Thus, a full diagnostic workup might not be what the patient is looking for in every case.

Hence the importance of the goals and preferences of the person who is actually suffering. I used to think, naively, that patients are typically not interested at all in diagnosis or the associated medical terminology. However, my research, as well as that of others, has found that this is not the case. Patients do want to know what they have, and this knowledge can be therapeutic. But since diagnosis, and even cure in some cases, does not necessarily correspond with symptomatic improvements, patients might be more interested in symptoms than in diagnoses, which goes against the grain of our current health culture.

If we can't necessarily cure all diseases according to a biomedical model, in which diagnoses exist in order to propel us, by hook or crook, toward a solution, can we make sure that every single disease can be treated according to the wants and needs of the patient rather than the algorithms of doctors' guidelines, applied wholesale?

This question is hard to answer for two reasons. First, the desires and preferences of human beings are rarely simple, are generally different from person to person, and tend to change over time. The second is that we do not know, for many illnesses, how best to tailor treatment according to those wishes and preferences.

This book is about these two complications: how to understand, as doctors and patients, the options available for common illnesses and how to bridge the gaps between imperfect medical evidence and the practical steps that might make these illnesses more bearable in our daily life.

How to Understand Outcomes That Are Relevant to the Patient

By now, you might have sensed a basic dichotomy—two different ways in which we can approach the experience of people with disease, understanding what it means to live with a disease and attempting to improve the condition.

One approach is through science—empirical research. The subfield known as patient-related outcomes research has never had so much attention in American health care. This is good. Patients' interests as individuals have been too long subsumed to what have been seen as the larger, and therefore more important, interests of populations as expressed in trials and doctors' guidelines.

More and more research articles delve into how patients define what is important to them in their life with a disease, how to collect and analyze that information statistically, how to make sure we are collecting the right information, and then how to disseminate and implement the research findings into interventions that can actually improve real life for people with disease. There is now a nongovernmental organization that promotes these aims, the Patient-Centered Outcomes Research Institute (PCORI). It was created by the same statute, the Affordable Care Act, that founded ObamaCare.

I do not know whether there has been a review of the effectiveness of PCORI's funding strategy—whether the funds disbursed have led to the furtherance of basic knowledge about patient-relevant outcomes or whether a link can be traced toward the funding of such research projects and actual improvement in patient health on a population scale.

Devotees of basic science might scoff at the simplistic nature of such proposed assessments. After all, the virtue of basic science is that we do not know beforehand how theoretical questions might lead to practical gains—nor, for that matter, are we competent in distinguishing what is theoretical and what is practical. If we take, for example, such wholesale changes in medical understanding as a unifying molecular mechanism of cancer (which was achieved through research funding) or—an earlier advance—whether depression is to be understood as predominantly a behavioral or social disease or as a complicated entity that is also affected by neuroscience, both molecularly and genetically, at what point do the so-called theoretical advances give rise to the practical?

Perhaps the PCORI is at the beginning stages of such a transformation, where we start understanding for the first time how patient-related outcomes might be placed at the center of medical research.

Or maybe such a quantitative approach to patient-centered care, pursued by the National Institutes of Health's top-down, large-scale model of research funding, is not the way to go. Perhaps we should instead take a qualitative route, collecting information on the basis of patient and provider narratives, as well as those of caregivers, so that we can extract themes that help us understand their experiences—the story, not the statistics.

To take an example from my work, my colleagues and I conducted qualitative research in order to understand the experiences of patients who have been diagnosed with prostate cancer of very low risk, according to criteria that show it is very unlikely for the cancer to grow or spread. Such people very often receive active treatment with surgery or radiation, even though such treatment for localized or very-low-risk prostate cancer is not associated with improved outcomes. In fact, it might be linked to adverse effects, as well as higher cost.[5]

The results of our analysis might help us understand how to approach the needs of people with low-risk prostate cancer. How do we know which patients, despite being in such a program that emphasizes monitoring over unneeded treatment, will leave the program and decide to have surgery or radiation?

We tried to understand patient experiences according to the qualitative approach. That is, we interviewed patients who have received treatment for such low-risk prostate cancer in order to understand their narrative together with the effects of the environment, the physician, and the person's attitudes, beliefs, and knowledge that impinge on their choices.

Using such methods, we found that the following was often true of patients in our sample: People have a fear of cancer and believe that any cancer is something that must, ipso facto, be removed root and branch, even if the very point of the program they are in is to monitor the disease without active treatment; people look to their physician for signals about the route they should take, interpreting any ambiguity as a reason to leave the program; patients are worried about the effects of monitoring the cancer without removing it; and a history of cancer in the family, even if not of the same variety, sensitizes people to their own prostate cancer, making them adjust the point at which they decide to have treatment.[6]

This method helped us identify important categories that might help explain why many patients with low-risk prostate cancer do not find it possible to participate over the long term in an active surveillance—that is, monitoring—program. This is useful for helping such programs better meet the needs of participants, understanding their anxieties and fears regarding cancer and helping them along from biopsy to biopsy as they navigate the uneven terrain of an unknown diagnosis.

However, this research cannot predict the behavior of a unique individual. This is where population research ends, whether quantitative or qualitative, and understanding a person begins, and this is the landscape of uncertainty that both provider and patient must deal with when living with a chronic disease. This landscape, in its different forms, is what we are exploring here.

PAYING ATTENTION TO THE PATIENT'S STORY

The problem with the difference between the experience of individuals and generalizable, empirical research obtained from populations is already well known. The plural of anecdote is data: we ignore the anecdote by subsuming it into a collection of data and calling the resultant evidence population based. How do we get back to the individual whose experiences and needs are revealed through the anecdote? What would it mean to pay attention again to the patient's narrative as she deals with chronic disease?

Attention to the patient's narrative is not new. Rita Charon of Columbia University is a pioneer in helping providers, and patients themselves, see that such stories must be told. In lectures, Charon says that the point of narrative medicine is not to understand the course of the patient's disease but to understand their individual experience. Thus, the narrative of the patient is meant to give the provider an insight, not as much into the care of the patient or the treatment as into the experience of what it is like to be a patient.

Understanding experiences can improve health care in all sorts of ways: by humanizing the relationship between doctor and patient; by making patients value their own experience; and by attuning the health care system to individuals rather than populations. Experiences, however, are not the same as care. Treating requires the participation not just of the person who is suffering but also of a second person who is outside of the patient's narrative. Understanding and narratives are not enough.

How can we bridge quantitative research into patient populations, qualitative research into the motivations of patients understood as individuals, the narratives of individuals conveying their experiences and apply them to the care of a given person with a given disease?

This book argues for a scientific, humanitarian, and patient-centered route to care all at once. I will use the term *individualistic care* in deliberate contrast with a current fashionable medical term: *individualized medicine*.

Individualized medicine refers to the use of genomic medicine, health care advances derived from genetic sequencing, for the benefit of the individual patient. This has become a scientific movement of importance, attracting funding and producing articles and advances with considerable speed. Individualized medicine has become a brand that is held aloft by the advocates of futuristic care. If only we knew how people reacted, with all their individual genomic predilections and dispositions, to a given medical intervention, we could tailor our medications to them and get them on the right doses.[7]

There has been considerable literature elucidating the influence of an individual's genome on the ways in which they react to warfarin (Coumadin), a particular kind of blood thinner. According to this literature, a provider would be able to tailor the dose of warfarin to a patient's genetic profile. The evidence that such individual tailoring will actually help patients live longer, avoid disease, or take medications at doses more appropriate for them, with a lesser burden of side effects, is at best incomplete.

We need to refresh our historical memories and go back to one of the founders of an integral and comprehensive look at care, George Engel, who promoted what is called *psychosocial medicine*. According to this outlook, the patient's care depends on an integration of a number of domains, from the individual's personality and psychological outlook to the social context in which he or she is embedded. It stands to reason, since each person's placement on their psychological and social axes is unique, that the individual's health status, future, problems, and outlooks should be unique as well.

How do we make sure that everyone is cared for in a way that respects their uniqueness, bringing what I call individualistic care to bear to every aspect of health care? It might seem that individualistic care might be more difficult in the case of common health problems, those that account for a significant part of health care expenditures, morbidity, and mortality, simply because they are the focus of worthy endeavors to improve care and a great number of guidelines promulgated by knowledgeable providers and backed by scientific evidence. These diseases are the ones on which medical science most reasonably focuses, for they are the new epidemics. Congestive heart disease, chronic pain, diabetes, psychiatric illnesses, HIV—these difficult medical and social conundrums inspire scientists to devise painstaking trials, which, if successful, give rise to effective treatments.

Interventions, however, no matter how effective they might be for the population, may not be appropriate for the individual. People, being who they are, might choose to make decisions that contradict the latest scientific evidence or the ballyhooed trial that has risen to the top of the guidelines issued by professional organizations. Both patient and provider might then run up against a frustrating divide: the patient wants what they want, and the doctor knows what the patient is supposed to want. How do they reconcile this difference?

Because these diseases are so widely discussed and studied, many doctors—and patients—labor under the misapprehension that there is a right way, and a wrong way, to participate in care for common problems. However, the fact of uncertainty must be recognized even for "run-of-the-mill" medical issues.

In the coming chapters, we will consider a number of prevalent (common) conditions in detail. For each condition, we will try to provide an integrated look at how the disease has been understood in the current biomedical paradigm of health care, how this paradigm has been changed in the era of evidence-based medicine and shared decision making, and, finally, how this synthesis might be further altered given our suggested approach of individualistic care. We will attempt to show, by way of conclusion, how individualized care can reinforce, not upend or revolutionize, evidence-based medicine and how it can map a research agenda for the coming century.

3

POVERTY

Making Decisions, Our Health System—and You in the Middle

Being sick is difficult; the difficulties of illness make other difficulties worse, and vice versa. Poverty both strengthens and complicates the connection between illness and life difficulties.

Yes, you might say, but poverty is not a disease. It modifies diseases. Is poverty really comparable to diabetes, hypertension, cancer, chronic pain, and all the other diseases discussed in this book?

I include it here because social determinants of health are not given enough attention in the individual interactions between doctors and patients. Poverty as a determinant of health is a focus of broad, deep, and long-term research among public health practitioners, but it doesn't get mentioned much when an individual doctor treats an individual patient.

How are doctors and patients supposed to approach a societal issue in the context of an individual's care? How can they try and improve care in the context of poverty?

Poverty is such a many-branched phenomenon, tied up with issues of race, education, and health literacy, that it might be controversial to address the economic aspects before the others. However, I will argue that addressing these economic realities is perhaps the most practical way for an individual patient to improve their care and to direct their doctor to options that matter most to them.

This does not mean that racial disparities are not vital to care. But their direct repair, though briefly addressed in the last chapter, are on the whole outside the scope of this book.

In this chapter, I want to emphasize the potential for our independent decision making, with the help of our doctors, in our health care encounters; understand how poverty gets in the way of that decision making; and talk about ways this can be remediated—without, of course, immediate infusions of cash (though I do believe in income redistribution).

On the one hand, we know that there are many ways in which too much health care is provided in our country's health system. There are too many medication prescriptions written, particularly for antibiotics,[1] too many laboratory tests done,[2] and too many advanced imaging procedures pursued,[3] all without clear evidence that they actually help. In short, there is overuse. Overuse costs money.

Unfortunately, good care costs money, too. There is an ongoing argument in the scientific literature regarding how care is distributed in the United States. Is the main problem overuse, too much care, or misuse and underutilization, the right care not given to the right people at the right time?

The right answer is probably the latter: a general diagnosis of our health-system problems is that we don't get the right treatments to exactly the right person just when and where they need it. And giving too much care is a subset of this problem.

The naive view would be to say that those people who can't afford such "overcare," whether through lack of insurance or lack of access, are actually escaping one of the worst characteristics of the health care system—the tendency to overtreat. If we have more access to health care (because of the expansion of Medicaid or ObamaCare or finding a job as the economy improves), will we be exposed to the worst part of the health care system, products and services we don't need?

This is a difficult question to answer. It requires interrogating the large literature on health services (whether people get what they need from the health care system and at what cost) and at the same time engaging in prophecy about what might happen to the health care system in the future.

It's clear that more health care is not necessarily better. But is some health care required? A 1998 paper in the *Annals of Internal Medicine* details the connection between access to care, quality of care, and results of care (outcomes).[4] It is difficult, but not impossible, to come up with something like an experiment showing that access to care can cause improved care. You would have to find a society that systematically denies care to a sector of the population, then allows that population to have care, and then measure the quality of that care before and after.

Conveniently enough, the United States has put that experiment into motion at least twice in recent decades. Medicare enabled previously uninsured people above the age of sixty-five to obtain care, and it appears that such care decreased mortality.[5]

In the second episode, going on even now, the Affordable Care Act (ACA) provided health care access for millions of Americans. The assumption, based in part on the previous experience with Medicare, is that such care will lead to decreased mortality and improved health in other areas.

I have a number of patients who go in and out of insurance. One of them, Mr. B, is a fifty-seven-year-old man with a complicated medical history, including kidney cancer (he has had one kidney removed), lung cancer (he has had part of his lung removed), multiple serious episodes of bleeding, and a heart attack. He is one of my most engaging and engaged patients, and I admire his ability to pursue his care even when he is between jobs. I asked him how he sets priorities and which care or medications he chooses to pursue when he has limited resources.

This is a conversation we have been pursuing over multiple visits, and one quote would not do justice to the ins and outs of all his deliberations. To summarize, however, he tells me that at some point he would like to have surgery for the aneurysm in his thoracic aorta that might kill him—but first, he wants to make sure that he has enough money saved up (even given his inconstant employment) to support his wife in case something terrible happens to him during the operation.

You might choose to prioritize differently. Prioritization—deciding which medicines or treatments to spend money on or take the time for rather than forgo, especially when one's time or resources are limited—might be relevant for everyone reading this book, no matter what your income strata or privileges are. But privilege, as described eloquently by an African American patient of mine, helps determine what one can or cannot do:

"My mother was a domestic worker. My father worked for Bethl'm Steel. Neither of them had any insurance. He died and they got insurance. Three thousand dollars. Eighty-eight dollars a month for her and the kids.

She didn't get any Social Security because of who she worked for. Three kids! Imagine if they had gotten sick. They never got sick. We never got sick! I think everyone should get health insurance. Why don't they want them to get health insurance?" she asked me.

"They don't like poor people," I responded.

"It's not their fault! I think everyone should have it."

This patient of mine, growing up and then while raising her family, tried to ensure, as much as possible, that she would not get sick since she was uninsured. Only recently, with the expansion of care through the Affordable Care Act, has she been able to get some of the care she needs.

One response of many of my patients, therefore, to their straitened circumstances is to prioritize care that keeps you from getting sick in the future. Of all the preventive-medicine strategies that doctors have proffered, the most effective might be those that can keep you from getting cancer. Depending on your time availability and your insurance coverage, the following cancer-preventive options might most sensibly be prioritized by someone with fewer resources.

Colon Cancer Screening

While several kinds of these screening tests have been found effective, possibly the most convenient involves testing for amounts of blood ("occult" blood) undetectable by the human eye, detected either by guaiac or by immunologic techniques. Both of these involve cards and are done at home, unlike a colonoscopy or sigmoidoscopy, which are done in a hospital setting, involve potential harms, and require inconvenient preparation (cleaning one's colon out beforehand) and a visit to the site where the procedure is done.

In addition, many colonoscopies are now accompanied by anesthesia, which requires the presence of someone to take you home afterward and monitoring while in the hospital, not to mention the presence of an anesthesiologist or nurse anesthetist to supervise the treatment itself.

Some of you might prefer a colonoscopy because you think it is more effective, but, as a matter of fact, the literature does not show that one mode of cancer screening is definitively better than the other. If you don't have much money and need to keep yourself healthy, this might be something to prioritize. Another kind of cancer screening it might be useful to think about is cervical cancer screening (if you have a cervix and have not had a hysterectomy), which has been shown to be one of the most cost-effective mortality reducers.

Some might say, however, that cancer screening is less important to a given individual—you reading this—than it is to a population. In other words, cancer screening is done from a public health perspective. Public health seeks to ensure the greatest health for the greatest number (or, depending on what philosophy you subscribe to, the great equality in health or to help the most vulnerable). However, you can legitimately claim as your greatest priority your own health and what matters to you. That is what makes the individual's health different from an algorithm.

If you are poor, how should you optimize your health? In this question, an assumption is concealed: if you are poor, your health is under your complete control. As a matter of fact, and history, we know that the American health care system is beset by various kinds of disparities that are not under an individual's complete control—hence their systemic nature. To instruct you, or anyone denied systemic privilege, to improve their lot assumes a level of individual agency that simply is not available to many.

Nevertheless, such agency is a cardinal future of autonomy, which everyone would like to arrogate to themselves. Thus we press on to ask the question: Even given the unfairness of the systems we are a part of, and even given our lack of resources to pursue the optimal care that is our due, how can we make things work in the best way possible without breaking the bank on our health care alone?

There are many examples of overuse in our health care system; though much attention has been devoted to it recently,[6] much overuse is still not sufficiently understood.[7] By turning the overuse problem on its head, we can address how those of us with the least amount of resources can approach the best health.

Avoid Over-the-Counter Preparations That Promise Health Promotion Without Evidence

You may have read the recent news that supplements sold in Walgreen's, Walmart, and other stores do not contain what they promise on the label.[8] What you also might not know is that even the supplements that do include what's on the label probably don't help, either.

An intelligent, educated friend recently wrote to me, asking what I thought about vitamins and what harms might be associated with them. I told her that, as far as I knew, there weren't all that many significant harms. Great, she said, and told me she was interested in taking them to boost her immune system. Unfortunately, there is no evidence that vitamins will do such a thing, but she is not alone in thinking this.

There must be something, people seem to think, to improve overall energy, something that can be bought or prescribed. There just isn't. And to the extent that these things cost money, not spending money on them might improve the balance between your own personal economic situation and your health. If supplements and vitamins don't eat up a big chunk of your income, cigarettes might. Or alcohol. Or other recreational substances.

COST-EFFECTIVENESS OF THERAPIES ON A LIMITED INCOME

The same questions about cost-effectiveness on a limited income can be applied to a lot of medical therapies. If you have high blood pressure, you might be taking a number of medications to treat hypertension, prescribed by your doctor. While a recent systematic review does show that treatment for hypertension reduces the rates of heart attack, stroke, and death, even in mildly high blood pressure (less than 160 over 100), treatment can encompass multiple forms, from medication to exercise to dietary changes. Any one of these treatments might be able to treat your mild blood pressure favorably, as we discussed in chapter 1; yet we don't know which treatment will best combine, for you, price and effectiveness—or cost-effectiveness, as the economists call it. There is a 1990 scientific paper that compares the cost-effectiveness of various pharmacological (medication) regimens for high blood pressure,[9] but this is different from knowing whether a medicine, diet change, or exercise will cost less money in the long run.

Such considerations can be important for every condition and every treatment: how much they cost you and how much they might cost you in the future. These questions are relevant to every disease I address in this book, but they are also relevant to larger issues about living your life, which are not necessarily fitted to the frame of medical decision making.

For example, will daily exercise, even given the inconvenience and possible conflict with other life responsibilities, be economically feasible in the long run while maintaining your health?

This goes back to a larger discussion, which has gone on for years in the philosophical and health care literature, about the difference between health and wellness. Do we seek the absence of disease or the fulfillment of all our capabilities in life? When we see health care professionals or embark on initiatives to improve our health, do we seek merely that—a lack of sickness—or a complete global level of function?

To answer a question with real attention to what you as an individual want, we should realize that such a question overlaps with the difficulties of achieving optimal health in a context of decreased resources.

If you define health as a complete, global wellness, then, if you are poor or part of a class afflicted by systematic disparities, it might be unrealistic to aspire to such a goal until the health care system, or the entire political system, is realigned toward greater equality. Telling ourselves to aspire toward a greater state of global wellness implies, perhaps unrealistically and even condescendingly, that we can somehow counteract the disadvantages of our situation and leap fully formed into a better life.

The person who just doesn't have enough money to make ends meet—who can't afford medications, who must choose between going to work and going to a doctor's appointment, who does not control his or her work environment and its impact on health—how is that person supposed to approach wellness in the sense of a comprehensive approach to his or her own existence?

But we can consider such a situation from another angle. If we cannot be expected to jump clear, by dint of self-activation, from economic or social difficulties imposed from without by systematic inequalities, we can use our situation to shed light on what health interventions might actually matter for us.

If we have limited access to resources—whether money, time, organization, control over our own work or family schedule—how can we best invest them in order to achieve global wellness?

This question is difficult to answer and is probably better approached by philosophers than patients or doctors. Given that we have finite money and time and limited opportunities, how should we structure our lives so that our health is optimized? Do we want to maximize the number of years we live or the quality of those years? Do we most care about reducing pain or making sure that we can live the way we want—that is, maintaining our "function" (however we would define that)?

PATIENT-RELATED OUTCOMES AND POVERTY

There is a large and growing field of research that addresses these questions regarding "patient-related outcomes."[10] This research is afflicted by the same problems that beset all health-related research that tries to address real-world issues: definitional issues and generalizability issues.

Definitional: How does one measure what outcomes are important to people? There are a number of indices out there, but they all measure slightly different things in various different ways. *Generalizability*: Patients are different, and we have different interests and needs. Any study is likely to address only a limited set of outcomes in particular categories of people.[11]

While philosophers spend a lot of energy trying to design or recommend the best way to live, it is unlikely that a given individual will be able to ask their doctor for an optimum "life design" to make their global wellness as high as possible.

Nevertheless, even in the absence of such incontrovertible priorities, we can identify some general guidelines that people can follow, continuing the advice that I have been giving in this chapter. For example, avoiding tobacco will save money and increase quality of life, as well as avoiding the increased risks of heart disease, lung disease, and cancer that tobacco can cause. A limited amount of alcohol consumption can cause pleasure, as Epicureans of all times have realized, but increased consumption can also increase the risk of high blood pressure, heart disease, and some cancers. Some illicit substances are widely recognized as deleterious to health—for example, cocaine and heroin—and others, while not free from harm, are becoming more widely used as part of the spectrum of substances that can make life more pleasurable.

Stronger still is the evidence behind the benefits of exercise, of meditation for anxiety and depression, and of a diet rich in fruits and vegetables. I am not making these recommendations in the voice of a clinical epidemiologist, who can ensure you (with more precision than long-term reliability in some cases) that changing the diet this way or that or adapting this or the other exercise program can reduce your risk of heart disease by so-and-so percent. No, I am making the claim that such life activities can increase happiness, are cost-effective, and do not appear to have any deleterious health effects. There are precious few things that are pleasurable and *won't* cause harm to our health, and this is one attempted list.

SYSTEMATIC FIXES: POVERTY AND HEALTH

With regard to the systematic problems of our health care system, most attention has been paid to disparities, which refer to differences in quality, cost, or access to care based on membership in a particular group, often due to systematic disadvantages that a particular group has borne. In the American context, this refers to the experience of African Americans and other minorities and, in particular, to the African American experience framed by slavery, institutional violence, and racism.

A multitude of fixes has been proposed to remedy disparities. Health disparities have rightly become a priority of our national health care system. However, possibly the most wide-ranging solution recently proposed for disparities in society at large, and the most virally distributed, was the call by writer Ta-Nehisi Coates for reparations to African Americans in order to redress the harms of institutional racism.[12]

Coates was not the originator of this idea, but he has brought it back into wide consideration. Though it is hobbled by numerous difficulties in theoretical conception and practical consideration, and it's likely not to meet with any success in the short term on the legislative front, it can provide food for thought regarding potential ways to make the health care system work for the poor and disadvantaged.

Reparations are just another means of income redistribution, giving support to those society has unjustly denied. But while reparations in their broadest form envision a large-scale effort that is potentially impracticable, health care reparations would be a more delimited, and potentially more practical, initiative.

How would redistributing health care resources work? Does it even make sense?

The first question is whether spending more or expending more health care resources (in the language of the economist) leads to better health care outcomes. This is surprisingly controversial. The past half decade, corresponding with the drafting, debate of, legislation, implementation of, and legal challenges to the Affordable Care Act, has coincided with sustained attention to the cost of health care in the United States, whether such cost constitutes "waste," and, if so, which parts of health care are wasted, exactly. This is a systematic problem that is relevant to the economy of the United States as a whole, as well as to our own personal economies. Even if we have health insurance, we still see some fraction of the cost. Even if we do not pay out of pocket or with our credit card for the health care procedures and treatments we are recommended, there is often still some amount of co-pay or at least an opportunity cost for the time we must take away from other things.

Given that health care costs in the United States are high and the quality—compared to that of other health care systems—is relatively low,[13] it has been proposed that much of this cost is due to waste. This claim has been buttressed by the maps of the *Dartmouth Health Care Atlas*,[14] which reach a surprising conclusion: health care services are provided in unequal ways across the United States in a distribution that does not seem to make much sense. Or, rather, if medicine is being provided in an evidence-based way to maximize effectiveness, one is hard pressed to understand why bariatric surgery should be performed seven times more often in Huntington, West Virginia, than in Winston-Salem, North Carolina.[15] Thus, it might make sense to say that the disproportionate cost/quality ratio of the American health care system is due to waste—too much spent for the wrong reasons.

That hypothesis seems plausible when examined at the level of the health care system as a whole. But studies on a different level—that of hospitals and patients—show a more complicated story. Some studies show no link between hospitals that spend more money on care and the quality of the care provided—that is to say, for example, patients' mortality and the outcomes of their various diseases. However, a recent comparison in California indicated that hospitals that spend more money on care deliver better outcomes, including for common diseases such as heart failure.[16] A recent complicated study done by health care economists based on data in New York State seems to indicate that patients from the same ZIP code delivered by ambulance to different hospitals (such ambulance assignments, as it turns out, are done nearly randomly) do better if they are brought to a hospital with higher costs.[17]

These data are confusing, and unfortunately they do not lend themselves to any one simple answer about the connection between systematic costs and your health.[18] Given the waste that is obvious in the health care system,[19] present in many instances of overtreatment and overuse, I personally find it difficult to believe that selecting the highest-cost doctor or hospital will, in general, lead to better care for yourself.

It is more likely that there are certain common conditions for which a certain minimal level of service, quality, and care is necessary for proper treatment, and a cost differential might indicate whether a health care facility reaches that minimum level. The question is: How do you know whether your doctor and hospital gets there in order to maximize the use of your limited resources? There are various means of public reporting—for example, websites that compare one doctor to another or one hospital to another.

The most reliable information is available through two sources: the federal government, which has mandated that hospitals[20] and doctors[21] provide certain kinds of information precisely for the purpose of such comparisons, or various journalistic concerns, which, taking a different tack, have tried to provide useful information to patients and other people who interact with the health care system for the sake of transparency— transparency regarding how much doctors and hospitals spend compared to the average in their categories, whether they accept pharmaceutical money,[22] and whether they have been involved in legal disputes. Such public reporting is a different animal, speaking to the concerns that any health care user might have about the unforeseen, harmful consequences of going to a doctor or hospital.

The different kinds of public reporting speak to the different ways that the health care system can lead to financial ruin. And while such ruin might not be frequent, it might be a way in which we can tailor our expectations of health care services to the evidence comparing doctors and hospitals to each other. A hospital that has had many patient complaints might not be worth our while economically. A doctor who has seen few patients from our ethnic group might not understand our limitations with sensitivity.

I wish this chapter were ending on a note of clearer advice or more straightforward evidence—that among poor people, or those with fewer resources, a particular course of action would lead to better health. The clearest conclusion that can be drawn is this: a certain minimal level of access to health care improves health. This minimal access includes doctors or hospitals that provide accepted treatment for acute and chronic conditions. From the research on overuse in the American health care system, we can speculate that the waste is due to treatments and technologies that are not needed (e.g., outlandishly expensive cancer medications that do not lead to proportional benefit) rather than necessary treatments for common conditions that must be delivered in order to reach some minimal standard of care.

Thus, since poor people and other disadvantaged groups, such as African Americans, are systematically denied equality of care by the U.S. health care system, there are certain initiatives that we as individuals can undertake, having to do with avoiding costly and untried interventions that do not improve our health, limiting expensive and health-destroying habits, and trying to find hospitals and physicians that meet our needs while limiting unnecessary cost.

Such initiatives on our part can only do so much to redress the disparities of our system. And thus, as others do, I consider it our duty as people seeking optimal health to advocate for a system that serves poor and rich equally, black and white, with the same attention to patients' health.

Advocacy is difficult for all of us, and I say that as someone whose profession implicates me in the very inequalities of the health care system. You would think that, as a provider, I would be involved in such advocacy. I can only say that I wish I were more effective in that regard. I hope that some of the examples I have given in this chapter might provide ways to think about not just our own health in the context of economics but also the health of others.

4

DEPRESSION

Medications? Therapy? None of the Above?

The gap between the medical language found in physicians' guidelines and the preferences of patients is especially noticeable in conditions that overlap with daily life experiences. For these conditions, it is not always apparent whether one person's departure from the norm is merely individual variety or a kind of disease that should be treated. Is obesity, by itself, a health condition to be diagnosed and treated, or is it merely greater-than-average weight, which is not incompatible with a healthy life?[1] There are people who catch more colds per year than others; is this an abnormality to be chased down and diagnosed or a natural example of statistical variation?

Mental health discussions are rife with such difficult distinctions. We know that feeling sad all the time might be due to challenges in our personal, work, or family lives; illness; financial stress; or unavoidable tragedy, which might strike us at any time. But there are people who feel sad without any outside provocation. Is their sadness due to their personality?

What makes depression different from sadness? There is obviously a huge literature covering this distinction, which I will not go into here.[2] But in deciding whether someone's (yours, a friend's, or a family member's) "depression" is something to be treated and, if so, whether to treat according to established medical technique or through some other means, I believe that three key factors need to be taken into account. Each of these helps illustrate the general points about chronic conditions and the difference between guidelines and preferences.

Before I mention these factors, I would like to tell the story of a patient in my practice (I am changing some of her identifying information to respect her privacy). She is a woman in her early fifties who works at a student center at a university in Washington, DC; she works the late shift, 7 p.m. to 2 a.m., when no one is around but the odd undergraduate studying or couples looking for a private corner. Most often, in my experience, people who work such hours have not necessarily chosen them willingly—and so it is with this patient. Three weeks before writing these words, she came into my office asking about a cold she had. I started to give her generic advice about the proper way to treat viral respiratory infections but realized she was looking crushed. I offered her some tissues, and she started to cry.

She comes from a large family, and most of her brothers and sisters (like so many in Baltimore whom I see as patients) are already dead. She feels alone a lot of the time. On this particular visit, she was crying because she got into a "spat" (she said, probably euphemistically) with her boss: "I'm not sure what happened; we had a meeting and I couldn't take it anymore, so I said something I shouldn't have."

She had come to me with a history of depression, but, as is so often the case, she didn't have any records from her earlier treatments, didn't remember which psychiatrist or psychologist she had seen, and didn't know what medications she had been on in the past. The only thing we both knew was that previously she had been "well controlled" on her depression medication (citalopram).

This phrase gets used a lot, and this is one of the key points to understanding the gap between depression as a subject of imperfect medical science and depression as it is lived—the gap between the "logic of decision making" and the logic of care that Annemarie Moll describes in her book *The Logic of Care*.[3]

What does it mean for depression to be controlled? The answer to this question goes back to the conflict between scientific evidence—how the questions are asked and answered and how the answers are presented—and how people live their lives. While data about populations can be collected and analyzed, sociologist Michael Polanyi made the observation that not everything about an individual can be known; every person knows "more than they can tell."[4] If you have depression, exactly what that diagnosis means for you might involve an individual experience that cannot be fully accessed by someone else.

This brings us to what "controlled" might mean for depression. If depression is a stand-in for a clinical term, defined according to the *Diagnostic and Statistical Manual of Mental Disorders* (*DSM-5*),[5] and its manifestations are certain carefully delimited sets of terms used in the research setting (symptom "flares"; *remission*, defined as an absence of symptomatic worsening), then those definitions can be applied to every individual equally. But if the experience of an individual cannot be necessarily reduced to these terms—without denying, of course, that these definitions can serve as useful guidelines—then we are thrown back on our own individual experiences as a way to guide our treatment.

Thus, if you or someone you love has depression and you are familiar with the two predominant treatment modalities, the story about the patient I mentioned above might be useful to you. When she saw me, crying, on the day after having a fight with her boss, she told me that she had stopped taking her depression medication—very common, as these medications are associated with significant side effects and are not effective 100 percent of the time, even in scientific studies—and did not think she needed to undergo therapy.

Now, according to the guidelines for the treatments of depression, the most effective options are medication or particular kinds of therapy (most particularly, cognitive behavioral therapy, though there is literature suggesting that other kinds of therapy might be as effective[6]). If someone were to reject these therapies—which this patient was—she might be characterized as "noncompliant" or "not participating in treatment." According to her own narrative, however, she was definitely taking steps to manage her depression. She took care of herself in this situation by discussing matters with her boss, asking for a refill of the medication to take again when she needed it, and finding people in her support system who could see her through her worsening symptoms. The definition of *control* was something that she herself determined in the moment.

If in our time together we had focused on the reasons why she had not taken her medication earlier, then she might not have felt free to tell her story about the progress of her symptoms and what might have caused them. Understanding the importance of the fight with her boss, rather than solely or mainly her compliance with medication treatment, was key to understanding the course of her symptoms.

The second key point to note—again, relevant to treatment in general for any physical or mental ailment—is that the effectiveness of treatments, determined in research studies, varies quite significantly in real life. The preponderance of the literature on treating depression finds, first, that the effectiveness of treatment depends strongly on the severity of depression, which makes intuitive sense. However, the severity of depression in real life can fluctuate from week to week, and this fluctuation is only "accessible"—that is, knowable—by the patient. Thus, a treatment that might be effective one week might not be as effective the next. [7]

Similarly, just as one primary care physician might not be as good as another, one psychotherapist or psychiatrist might not be right for a given patient. Alexandria Quillen, a twenty-three-year-old woman in Newnan, Georgia, with chronic mental health problems, talks about a successful relationship with a therapist this way, in an interview with me by e-mail in August 2015:

> In 2013, I was running out of steam. The more I tried to understand everything . . . I just couldn't. This was the year that I got with a very gifted psychiatrist who cared for me like a human being should. She never labeled me as a challenging or difficult patient—she helped me to find myself. I went through intense therapy and constantly had my buttons pushed in order for me to make progress.

She acknowledges that there is always uncertainty associated with her diagnosis, treatment, and care, but the uncertainty has as much to do with the unknown quality of the provider she sees as with the nature of her diagnosis and treatment: "[My uncertainty isn't exactly] about my prognoses but the professionals that give the prognoses, the type of care I will receive every time I reach out. I don't want to feel that the health care provider is holier than me. I want their actions to never let me forget that we both bleed red blood."

Finding a therapist you can stick with or a psychiatrist who takes your insurance can be fiendishly difficult and can make the difference between stable care over time and scrambling, month after month, to find someone who can refill your medications or provide you with therapy. Although in 2008, even before the Affordable Care Act, parity in coverage was legislated for physical health and mental health services, this does not guarantee parity in pricing, quality, or access. That is, insurance companies can charge more for mental health services than for other health services.

Access to mental health services is difficult at best, and in some areas of the country, it is almost nonexistent.[8]

All of this information converges on a suggestion that is at cross-purposes to the prevailing assumption of the American health care system: that people must see specialists for the various maladies that afflict them. Specialists are very important, of course, and no less so in mental health, particularly in cases where we haven't found a treatment that works for us or we are extremely ill (e.g., with thoughts of suicide, hallucinations, or other disturbing symptoms that we can't control) or we have a preexisting relationship with a mental health provider who serves our needs.

Many people diagnosed with depression have milder symptoms,[9] and if those of us with depression can be trusted to track our own symptoms, judging a treatment's effectiveness by our own lights—while having recourse to the care we want when we need it—then perhaps the provision of mental health care could be made more equal, convenient, and effective. In other words, we ourselves, the ones suffering from depression, can take care of our own symptoms together with the help of a primary care provider, without necessary recourse to a psychiatrist. In the majority of cases, this will be sufficient.

In the majority of cases, this will be sufficient. If you have depression or know someone who does, this advice might seem foolhardy. But you must correctly understand what I am suggesting here. I am not saying that someone with depression should divorce himself or herself from all care. As I broached in the introduction, and as should be evident throughout this book, one of the ways we can improve our health is recourse to care when it is necessary. The foundation of the benefit that a doctor brings a patient for a chronic condition is not predominantly the technological armamentarium, nor pharmacologics, nor batteries of tests, but rather the ability to provide a relationship that, serving as an outside perspective, can help answer our questions and provide guidance when we know things are worse—as Alexandria Quillen puts it, doctors "deal with the questions and fight the battle with me."

Given that a doctor, even a primary care doctor, only sees his or her patients every once in a while and is not continuously present in our lives, we must figure out how to deal with chronic conditions when we are outside the doctor's office.

We have several choices. On the one hand, we can accept the course of treatment that we discuss in the doctor's office. Ideally, as I discussed in my first book, *Talking to Your Doctor*,[10] this visit would be characterized by good communication, involving a dialogue between people who see each other as people, bleeding the same blood, as we heard Alexandria say. On the basis of such communication, including a discussion of treatment options, risks, and benefits and your preferences and values, you will make a decision on a course of treatment.

But "following a treatment regime for depression" is basically, given the demands of real life, strongly dependent on what real life allows, what treatments work with our needs as individuals, what varieties of care work for us, and how we understand the course of our disease. Indeed, even among those diagnosed with depression, there might be various opinions about how, or whether, "depression" differs from a change in mood that is part of normal life.

We should not automatically assume that meeting with our doctor about depression will provide us with a treatment regimen for depression that we can then follow. Consider the findings of studies of medication treatment for depression, which find, in general, that they are 50 percent or so effective (keeping in mind the fact that these studies are limited to the healthiest sectors of the population). Moreover, the evidence for depression medication itself is beset by all sorts of difficulties. Few studies compare medications in the same class or therapy with medication to therapy by itself or medications of different classes.

So what can we get out of seeing a doctor (or other care provider) regularly if following a determined care regimen might not work for us? For depression, there are several benefits. First, in a regular care provider, be it a doctor or nurse, we find a reliable outside source to help us track our own symptoms. Sometimes in the midst of a chronic condition, as the multiple stressors of life intervene, we cannot achieve enough distance from ourselves to know what is our own depression, what is something else (e.g., fatigue or chronic pain), and what are the normal ups and downs of life.

Alexandria shares with us a similar situation from her life.

> Many times, I question my diagnoses—I cycle between acceptance and denial. Are they sure this isn't just hormone related? Maybe I am not mentally ill. What if my flank pain isn't the cause of trigger points but kidney problems? Maybe I have kidney disease, just like my

father. What if my chronic pain is coming from a detectable problem and isn't just a syndrome? Few doctors have been willing to deal with my questions and fight the battle with me. They become frustrated with me and give up. I ask a ton of questions, and I am involved in my treatment. I refuse to follow health recommendations blindly. I have a mind and I am very intelligent—few doctors respect me for who I am and don't treat me like a symptom rap sheet.

Perhaps the doctors are frustrated with Alexandria's changing understanding of her condition because, like so much else about the chronic conditions we discuss here, it does not fit on the tracks of the confined definitions according to which physician guidelines are devised and scientific trials conducted. But we, and our doctors, need to realize that our symptoms will never neatly fit those described in the rigid confines of such trials. Thus, with the help of our care providers, we need to keep track of how we are feeling.

Second, follow-up with a physician can help us realize the available treatment options and, in the best of circumstances, the limitations of the scientific evidence. Consider table 4.1, which describes, briefly, the gaps of the evidence regarding depression treatment. It is a summary of what is not known, what scientists call research gaps.

Since there are so many unknown questions, one can reasonably ask what we can actually do to treat our depression. We might feel hopeless or confused that nothing can be said to work the same way for everyone. We might be frustrated that claims made for medications do not seem to

Table 4.1. Optimal Treatments for Depression: Gaps and Questions

1. In which groups of people (ethnic, racial, income) is therapy better than medication?

2. Can therapy be better than medication in some phases of the illness but not in others?

3. In which kinds of people with severe depression is the net effect of medication deleterious and not helpful?

4. In which people with mild depression can the disease resolve on its own without treatment? Which treatments (apart from medication and therapy) can lead to such resolution?

5. Does the cost-effectiveness of therapy (compared to medication) differ with the severity of depression?

6. When patients guide their own therapy without regard to physicians' guidelines, do they improve faster?

7. Do primary care providers help depression treatment as much as specialists?

hold up or be applicable to us as individuals. What, then, should our next step be?

Practically speaking, obviously, the following suggestions only apply to people who aren't very sick with their depression. Just to get out of the way what shouldn't need to be said: if you are so ill as to be thinking about or planning suicide or to put yourself or others in danger in some way, then you should seek care immediately, preferably in an emergency room.

As obvious as this advice sounds, the fact that it is necessary points to something important about depression treatment. Depression is what psychiatrists call *ego-dystonic*: it does not feel good. If you have ever suffered from depression—and there are, of course, many eloquent expressions of this feeling in the literature—you know that it is not something you want to continue. Yet there are multiple cases in which people with depression do not receive the care they need or encounter a denial (on their own part) that the disease needs treatment at all. This is very different from acknowledging that we have no single best treatment, but it is related. How so?

Often when we are dealing with a disease, we come to a doctor expecting an answer. We think that he or she has a handle on what the evidence is—there must be some answer out there to tell us how to proceed in our case. Yes, there are conflicting studies, but medical training together with a knowledge of us, the patient as an individual, provides the key to tunnel down through all of the uncertainty to the real truth of greatest effectiveness.

Scientifically speaking, there is no such truth in depression. The number of outcomes (results or treatment) that might matter to one person are different from those that might matter to another. From a public health perspective, we can even argue about which is more important: the number of deaths saved by preventing suicide or the disability and life disruption associated with untreated depression.

From an individual perspective, different people find different things about depression most disruptive. Is stabilizing mood most important, even given the change to personality and the harms of medication that such treatment might involve? Is addressing the disruption to family and work life most important? Can we entrust our symptoms to a therapist with the associated inconvenience, loss of privacy, and cost? Again, there is no single answer to such questions.

This single answer also will not be found through the newest scientific research. This might be interpreted as an antiscientific remark. It is not. The relationship between science and medicine is complicated, and it is worthwhile to make some distinctions. It is impossible to derive any consistent definition of what is, or isn't, "science." One can, however, talk about kinds of science that are or are not relevant to patient care. Indeed, for the sake of human knowledge, every kind of search for knowledge is valuable. But the relevance for health care is not the same for every branch of science. To take a relevant recent example, in an article in the *New York Times*, current advancement in imaging technology was cited as a potential treatment for depression. [11]

Leave aside whether the new research on functional imaging in depression shows a potential route to clinical improvements somewhere down the line—it might very well be true—and focus on the present. In the treatment of depression, these fancy images provide nothing to help an individual person, except in very rare cases in which a previously undiscovered abnormality in the brain might be causing mood disorders (e.g., a cancer or unrecognized seizures). But the belief that science can help the individual directly and predictably on the basis of its discoveries is unwarranted. Brain imaging does not lead to the treatment of depression but perhaps to a sense, in a minority of people, of what is underlying the symptoms—if any structural cause can, in fact, be pointed to.

What science can do for us when we suffer from a chronic condition is to outline the contours of the possible. What treatments have been shown to improve depression in clinical trials? What are the kinds of therapy that work? But perhaps even more immediately useful to us as individuals suffering from depression is research on the ways in which health care services can best be used.

Even if advanced brain imaging—for example, MRIs, which show how the brain is functioning in the moment—were able to diagnose depression earlier or tendencies toward the development of depression later in life, the question would be: How does this relate to the treatment of a given individual? Does finding out a potential diagnosis earlier help matters or merely attach a name to something that can't be helped in the early stages anyway? (Can depression be treated even before it is associated with evident symptoms?) If that brain imaging is truly indicative of depression, are our treatments good enough to make early diagnosis worthwhile?

Health services research examines how the various parts of health care fit together: who receives what kind of care, how it is received, at what cost, and with what results. Such research shows us that undergoing testing for depression very much depends on the environment in which it is given. If depression is more common in a group of people, then looking for depression in that group might be more effective—but only if there are treatments that help. In an environment in which depression, if present, is less severe, looking for it might not improve the health of a population. [12]

If we are in a situation in which we need the infrastructure that a primary care provider, in concert with a mental health practitioner, might provide, obtaining regular care for our depression might be right for us. Regular care would enable us to discuss a potential medication regimen, keep a close eye on the harms that would likely follow starting a medication (because all medications involve harms), decide what should be the right balance between medication therapy and psychotherapy, and understand the interaction between psychosocial factors (i.e., the stressors and pressures of life) and these other kinds of treatment. You, together with your doctors, would be able to determine what trial period would be necessary before pursuing such treatments on your own.

Pursuing treatments on your own would not mean abandonment by your doctor but working together with him or her in order to find potential routes to improvement. The practical barrier to depression treatment coordinated and controlled by those suffering from the disease is the fact that a doctor's agreement is required for many of the available forms of treatment. For example, medications are given by prescription only, and psychotherapy is often difficult to access and, once it is secured, is often not covered by insurance. But if you find someone who might be able to empower you to undergo treatment on your own recognizance, you might find a combination that works better than treatment by someone who is not able to give credence to your experience.

The discussion of depression here might seem suspiciously commonsensical: ask your health care provider what works; if you are not seriously ill, use your own thought processes and trial and error in order to figure out what is right for you since the scientific literature is not reliable enough to determine a unique course of treatment for a given individual. You might, again, need to have access to a doctor who can provide you with that treatment, which is why alternative and complementary techniques are certainly worth trying. Common sense should be the rule here because many inflated claims are often made for the importance of breakthrough new technologies in the treatment of depression. In addition to the advanced imaging mentioned above in the *New York Times*, we have heard—on various occasions—that smartphones with installed apps can help people "know when they're depressed" or supplement the care of a health care provider.

Unfortunately, if you have difficulty accessing a doctor or nurse or treatment for your depression, you might also be the sort of person (due to your life circumstances or race) who could have difficulty accessing such an app. If you are provided an app that is tailored to the phone or computer available to you, will it help you more than writing down your symptoms on a piece of paper? This is not to deny that an app will make it easier to keep track of your symptoms, but the scientific literature linking technological solutions to better treatment of depression might not be there yet.

What is the hope that you can hold onto for yourself or your family member as you make your way through life with depression? If, as I said, the evidence supporting any given treatment for depression is so imperfect as to be unimpressive and treatments themselves are difficult to access and pay for, what is the route forward?

As with so many other chronic conditions, it depends on how severe your depression is. Obviously, if you are suffering from depression that makes it difficult to work, live, take care of your kids, or get out of bed, then by all means an intensive course of treatment is necessary, if only to receive help in the sustained fashion that you will need to survive the worst parts of the illness. This might involve inpatient treatment in a hospital, intensive outpatient treatment in a facility, or frequent visits with a mental health or primary care provider whom you trust. It is important to note that both doctors and nurses can aid in depression treatment, and the literature does not seem to indicate that one kind of provider is better than another. [13]

What I would like to suggest here is more relevant for people with mild or moderate depression. Sure, there are study-based definitions in the scientific literature of what makes mild and moderate differ from severe, but in essence these are distinctions that have to made by you as an individual. If you are able to fulfill your life responsibilities and function according to your lights, but depression is disruptive to you, then self-management of your symptoms might be a practical route for the reasons I have already mentioned: the lack of strong evidence that pharmacological treatment (medication) is better than other sorts of treatment for depression; the ability to implement independently, given a support structure, the beneficial elements of cognitive behavioral therapy; and the necessity of integrating depression treatment into one's own life.

This does not mean that recourse to a provider would not necessarily be of no use. There will be times when a knowledge base is needed: What medications are available? What therapies do you trust? Is there an underlying medical disorder that needs to be ruled out here? But these are more in the nature of general needs for support and advice rather than the armamentarium of medicine, based on the dictates of a supposed science, which have fixed the direction of depression treatment for so many up to now.

This route to the self-treatment of depression has to do with the notion of *phronesis*, practice, which has lately been applied to the work of physicians. But I think it can usefully be applied to the experience of ordinary people, too. Phronesis is a kind of practical moral wisdom. An example from Aristotle is described in the *Stanford Encyclopedia of Philosophy*: a distinction between kind children and kind adults. Kind children know to be nice but lack the practical wisdom to implement this knowledge.

> Adults are culpable if they mess things up by being thoughtless, insensitive, reckless, impulsive, shortsighted, and by assuming that what suits them will suit everyone instead of taking a more objective viewpoint. They are also, importantly, culpable if their understanding of what is beneficial and harmful is mistaken. It is part of practical wisdom to know how to secure real benefits effectively; those who have practical wisdom will not make the mistake of concealing the hurtful truth from the person who really needs to know it in the belief that they are benefiting him. [14]

We can understand self-care with the help of this concept of phronesis. When a person is able to take an objective viewpoint of their own care in order to secure real benefits, they will be able to face the truth about the course of their symptoms and take the necessary steps to remedy matters.

In depression in particular, speaking of practical wisdom is difficult. It is very easy, given societal stigma toward the mentally ill, to blame the person for his or her condition. If we approach self-care as a practice, converting the wisdom we have stored about ourselves and our bodily processes into practical action, any failure might be placed at our own feet. This is one of the greatest fallacies of medicine as currently practiced, which reinforces the disparity associated with common conditions: if we, ordinary people, did everything "right," somehow we would manage to achieve health. Any deviation from health must somehow be our own fault.[15] If the evidence for the treatment of depression is incomplete and the available treatments imperfect, where does the truth lie? Surely we cannot be expected to treat ourselves? What if we fail?

Failure happens, and there is no shame in it. While failure is painful and an obstacle, it need not be fatal or destructive to future self-treatment. Failure comes with the treatment of any disease. Certainly, with depression, one must take care that the most dangerous chasms of the disease are avoided. As I mentioned above, the worst outcome associated with depression is suicide attempt and completion—that is not a failure we should countenance. But in the vast regions of mild and moderate disease, we can realize that the scope of failure we might commit in self-care, when possible, is comparable to the mistakes we would make when following the treatment recommendations of a doctor.

What would a self-care of depression look like? There are several elements, all commonsensical and none originally thought up by me. In fact, they are based on tried-and-true techniques developed by psychotherapists, the bread and butter of their practice. They are also applicable to many of the chronic conditions discussed in this book: keeping a diary of symptoms; making sure that friends and family are available to support you; ensuring that you participate in regular activities (physical, cognitive, and emotional) that have been shown to reduce symptoms of depression;[16] and knowing where to go and whom to call if your symptoms become seriously worse.

This all assumes, of course, that you have access to a support structure. What happens if you don't? What if you are on the margins, whether financially or racially or with regard to your sexual or gender orientation? What are you supposed to do? Some of the advice above might apply to you, but, unfortunately, given the disparities of our system, it might not. Thus, this is where my easy advice stops and my hard advice begins. If self-care as moral practice is at all a possibility, and I think it is a crucial part of care for these conditions as more and more we recognize the imperfection of medical evidence, then it has to be made possible for everyone equally. And that means advocacy for those who do not have access to infrastructure and support. Depression is marked by stigma, and stigma can only be relieved through a change in culture. Knowing that depression is not to be treated the same way for everyone might imply the necessity of a way to recognize the individuality of those who deal with the disease.

Imperfect evidence does not, in short, mean that those with depression have to go it alone, but we need to make self-care possible for everyone so that each person can figure out what works for him or her as an individual.

5

HIGH BLOOD PRESSURE

Where Is the Limit?

"The doctor told me I have high blood pressure." We've said it our-selves or heard a loved one say it to us. But what does that mean, and what should we do about it?

The story of high blood pressure is a story of a disease that came into existence bit by bit over decades, has spawned a billion-dollar industry and dozens of medications to treat it, and is overtreated in some while untreated in others. How did hypertension get this way? If we know that people's blood pressure is high and potentially related to increased rates of heart attack and stroke, shouldn't it be easy enough to decide to treat it and reduce those diseases in the population at large?

The current chapter of the story starts with the realization that about three-quarters (73 percent) of all those diagnosed with high blood pres-sure take medication for the condition, while only 50 percent of all those with high blood pressure have it "controlled" through such treatment.[1]

This has been adduced as evidence that hypertension is "undertreated" and that our system should be tasked with getting more Americans to take medication for high blood pressure.[2] If we could only identify all those people with high blood pressure, get them to a doctor, get that doctor to prescribe them medication, and get them—somehow—to take their medi-cation, then we would prevent a whole lot of disease.

Undoubtedly this is partially true. Among those whose high blood pressure has not been diagnosed, and undoubtedly some of you are reading this, there are those who would benefit from pharmacological treatment—taking medication.

But there are also those who would not benefit from such treatment. Medications are always associated with potential harms. Doctors are not good at discussing these harms with us. Either they disclose too much, listing every little possible side effect that can happen in any universe and scaring us half to death, or they gloss over potential harms with a vague mention that "everything will be fine." If everyone were on treatment, some of those people would be exposed to medication-related harms.

Some more of the theoretically "untreated" population with high blood pressure would have mild hypertension, which is defined in a number of studies as a systolic (top number) of 160 or below and a diastolic (bottom number) of 100 or below. The most recent systematic reviews of the scientific literature, which use particular algorithms to review, select, and pool results of medical studies, show that treatment of mild hypertension does benefit people, leading to fewer heart attacks and strokes. It is unclear whether those with mild hypertension who end up being treated will see benefits to their longevity or whether, even with fewer events related to blood vessel disease (i.e., fewer strokes and heart attacks), they will die of something else after living as long as they would have otherwise.[3]

In these studies, *treatment* does not refer only to treatment with medications. To be clear, the systematic review I am referring to above, which pooled the results of a number of scientific studies, showed that treatment of high blood pressure did lead to lower rates of various blood-vessel-related illnesses. But a number of other sorts of effective treatment are also available. Thus, if millions of Americans are in fact "undertreated" for high blood pressure, would they be better off, all in all, if as many of them as possible were treated with medications, given that estimates of harms for these medications, as they are used in daily practice, are hard to come by?

Further, if many of us were treated for blood pressure, what would be the best combination of treatments for us? That is, how many of us should ideally be on a pharmacological (medication) treatment and for whom should the best treatment be, instead, a change in the way we live our lives, without recourse to medication?

I don't know of any scientific study that attempts to estimate what the optimal distribution of blood pressure treatment is in a population. On the one hand, there are various types of blood pressure treatment: pharmacological treatment with medication, exercise, change in diet, quitting smoking, limiting alcohol consumption, reducing stress, weight loss, general relaxation techniques. On the other hand, there are various types of people (those with diabetes, preexisting heart disease, and kidney disease) for whom tighter blood pressure control is widely recommended. Then there are people who are more or less healthy. Finally, cutting across these categories, there are people with all of the complications that life presents: insufficient income and housing (all the inconveniences and barriers that go along with poverty), a low familiarity with all of the jargon and bureaucracy of health care, caregiving responsibilities for others in the family, low English proficiency, struggles with substance use or abuse, inability to access health care or afford medications.

Imagine a huge database. On one side, all of the blood pressure treatments would be lined up; on the other side, the different groups of people and their—our—difficulties. In each cell of the database, you would find some sort of number or perhaps a narrative describing how you would feel on that combination of treatments. Only the cells—in the best possible world—would not be how you would feel just at one point in time but your condition over years. And the rows on one side would represent not just individual treatments but also every possible combination of treatments with every possible combination of doses and mixtures of medication treatment, lifestyle treatment (e.g., through exercise), and other treatments or trying something for a few years and then trying nothing at all.

The database is difficult to visualize and admittedly implausible because it is completely unlike how we experience our medical care. We do not slot ourselves into one or another cell but somehow, in the interstices of life and our experience of disease, manage to fit in our treatment. Given the delay that is often present between when we realize a problem to be present, when we see the doctor, and when we start treatment, and then given the frequent inability to note how our symptoms have responded to treatment, we might not even know if the medication we are taking (assuming it is a medication that we have chosen) is helping.

But this algorithmic, spreadsheet model of health care is exactly how some doctors see guidelines, the sets of recommendations that physicians and other health care providers are encouraged to follow.

Physicians and patients are encouraged to follow algorithms for obvious reasons. First, it can improve care for entire populations. It really is true that getting as many people as possible on treatment for high blood pressure can reduce rates of heart attack and stroke. Thus, considering the entire population as one population, we would know the right thing to do: prescribe medication for as many people diagnosed with high blood pressure as possible and make sure that they are actually taking it.[4]

If only it were that simple! This is the distinction between public health and individual health, between concerns of the public at large, or society, and your individual concerns and needs. Everybody, ideally, would be on blood pressure treatment, but then again, you are not "just everybody." We are all our own unique personalities, lives, and difficulties.

Many of us might prefer to prevent heart attack, stroke, kidney disease, and other consequences of high blood pressure. But some of us might have other priorities.

Mr. D may provide an illuminating example to help us understand our own priorities and where they might differ from algorithms based on population-level outcomes. He works at Johns Hopkins, as do I. But while I have a relatively cushy job as a doctor, he works in the operating room (OR) as a so-called service associate—he helps clean the OR between procedures, a stressful responsibility.

Mr. D takes three medications for blood pressure, some of which you yourself might be taking: amlodipine, a calcium channel blocker; a diuretic (water pill), hydrochlorothiazide; and an angiotensin-converting-enzyme (ACE) inhibitor. The most common side effects associated with these medications, from the first to the last on the list, are leg swelling, dizziness and electrolyte abnormalities (even falls in the older population), and kidney damage or cough.

But, of course, high blood pressure is not his only problem. He has terrible depression and anxiety, possibly due to the time when, on his stoop in Baltimore, heading into his house, a man with a gun threatened him. Mr. D has a stress disorder that has never been treated due to the stigma attached to mental health problems, the difficulty involved in taking time off from work to receive treatment, and his disinclination to take additional medications if he can avoid it.

From this stress disorder, or possibly existing before it, he has to deal with severe depression and anxiety, which manifest themselves in episodes of panic. These episodes can happen in the middle of the workday and are characterized by pounding heartbeat, shortness of breath, headache, trembling, and a feeling of doom. Since he works in a health care environment, at these times, reasonably enough, his colleagues tell him to check his blood pressure. Then he finds his blood pressure elevated, which makes him even more anxious, and the cycle continues. Finally, his manager sends him to occupational health. When his blood pressure is checked there, this again makes him anxious, as his ability to return to work is dependent on their blood pressure reading, and he is surrounded by a number of nurses and other assistants checking his blood pressure all at once.

So he comes to see his doctor—me—to ask what he should do about his blood pressure. What would you do if you were in Mr. D's shoes?

Would you first treat your panic disorder, your depression, or your anxiety, knowing that it would mean an additional investment in time (even if you did find a psychologist who might take your insurance), or would you take additional medications? You might be reluctant to tell your occupational health office about it, because then they would be unlikely to let you return to work.

Mr. D decided to take an extra dose of his blood pressure medications so that he would be allowed to return to work. As we have listed above, one potential side effect of the so-called ACE inhibitor he is taking is a decrease in kidney function. Thus, due to the pressure to return to work, he has placed himself in possible jeopardy.

What is the root cause of his worsened blood pressure and incomplete blood pressure control? And what can be done about it?

There are many things going on here at once: work stresses, untreated psychiatric illness, previously existing high blood pressure, anxiety due to the act of checking blood pressure. None of these can be fixed all at once. But we should start with something.

Here are the choices I made when talking with Mr. D about the best route to start with.

First and foremost, I recommended to Mr. D that he address his mental health issues. Many people with high blood pressure also have psychological or psychiatric diagnoses.[5] This is not surprising, because the sources of high blood pressure—in essence, blood pressure outside the norm—track closely with the sources of mental health problems and psychological disease—in essence, disruptive mental patterns outside the norm. People who have depression and anxiety tend to have high blood pressure as well because of the inequities of our societal design. Those with high blood pressure tend to have high levels of stress, which predispose them to these mental health conditions.[6]

This is not to say that every person with high blood pressure necessarily has mental health diagnoses as well. Far from it. Or that everyone with a psychiatric or psychological diagnosis suffers from high blood pressure. Merely that when we consider our magical, optimal, comprehensive database, with the treatments of high blood pressure on one side and the type of people on the other, and when we consider the categories any one of us might fall into, we have to understand that there are multiple dimensions extending out of the page—and one of them is mental illness.

I think it unlikely that Mr. D will receive the treatment he needs. Perhaps he doesn't feel that it is right for him. Perhaps he does not have access to reliable care. Or perhaps he does not have the stability of income and employment necessary to take time off in order to see a provider. It is likely that he conceives of his mental health issues in the same way many other people do: as a problem due to his physical health issues rather than the other way around. "I get stressed when my blood pressure is up," he has told me a number of times.

If he is not in a situation to obtain regular and effective care for his depression and anxiety, then perhaps the next best treatment for him would be to find some sort of relaxation technique that he can implement in his home or work.

But this ignores the social setting of his disease. It is impossible for him to reduce the level of his stress when he is in a stressful work environment, and that stress is compounded when he makes his way home. (In his case, his sister recently suffered a house fire, so he took care of several extra members of his family who had to stay in his apartment. Obviously this is his own particular story, but there are many with such stressors in their lives.)

Let us take a step back for a broader view of what is necessary to treat hypertension: understanding the social determinants of health.

The physiologist and physician Rudolf Virchow said,

> Medicine is a social science and politics is nothing else but medicine on a large scale. Medicine as a social science, as the science of human beings, has the obligation to point out problems and to attempt their

theoretical solution; the politician, the practical anthropologist, must find the means for their actual solution. [7]

We know that, certainly in the individual case of Mr. D, his social circumstances, which in turn are deeply affected by the structure of society, have a lot to do both with the blood pressure as he feels it now and with the options available to him to potentially lower it, as well as with his conception of the benefits and harms of participating in various kinds of blood pressure treatment. Just as in the case of those of you who may have been diagnosed with high blood pressure, Mr. D must decide between stable employment, necessary to support his family and relatives, and the stress it occasions him.

Paradoxically, Mr. D's job in a hospital makes it more likely that his anxiety and high blood pressure will go hand in hand. Whenever he feels anxious, he goes to one of his colleagues or an anesthesiologist who works in the same operating room that he does, and they suggest that he check his blood pressure. This might seem like a reasonable course of action. However, except for the circumstance in which someone is changing the dose of his or her blood pressure medicines, trying to find the doses at which pressure is optimally controlled, I know of no evidence that indicates it is helpful for someone to check his or her blood pressure multiple times a day. Thus, Mr. D's health care colleagues are trying to be helpful but are also enabling his worry and obsessive checking of his high blood pressure, which makes things worse.

So how often should Mr. D check his blood pressure?

It depends on the reason he has for checking it. The diagnosis of hypertension, according to commonly used guidelines, requires repeated readings. [8] More recent literature, however, indicates that blood pressures checked at home by patients can be more accurate than those checked once or twice during a visit to the clinic. And the gold standard for blood pressure checking is now more and more understood to be ambulatory blood pressure monitoring, in which one wears the monitor in question, a box on the chest with a blood pressure cuff, for twenty-four hours. [9]

I think getting this concentrated burst of information—the entire run of blood pressure readings, sleeping and waking, eating and working, walking and at rest—could help Mr. D control his blood pressure as much as frantically checking it at work every day. And perhaps such monitors should be available for more of us.

If one route to improving his blood pressure control is controlling the stress of his environment, or at least recognizing the stress and doing something about it (through therapy, family support, relaxation techniques, or the like), and another is checking his blood pressure in the more accurate way, still another route, and probably the most important, is recognizing the potential harms of the medications that he might be prescribed for high blood pressure.

Every medication, every treatment, involves harm. When we go to the doctor, we expect a discussion of the risks and benefits attached to a particular treatment, but we might not think about the best way to do this beforehand. Do we need a list of all of the benefits and all of the risks? The most common in each category? The most salient benefits and most nightmarish risks? And how do we balance the two categories when they include different kinds of members? That is, how do we compare a decreased risk of heart disease or stroke to an increased risk of dizziness?

I would like to suggest, based on the experience of my patients, a somewhat heterodox, if not entirely new, approach to the treatment of hypertension. Pick a numerical goal with your doctor and aim to get there *only if* you do not find that the medications somehow pose a burden to you. There are plenty of methods to quantify the balance between benefits and harms, or pluses and minuses, of medication treatment. Decision trees can attach numbers to each potential choice branch; sophisticated computer programming can "gamify" the process of choice; decision aids can walk people through the alternatives of various courses of treatments. Yet, at bottom, the most consequential choice in the case of treatment for hypertension on the basis of medication is whether to take a given medication.

I will take a moment here to address an important new study of blood pressure control via medication that has received a lot of press just as this book is in the final stages of preparation. Called the SPRINT study,[10] this trial randomized about nine thousand people aged fifty and above to two kinds of blood pressure target: one more intensive, where a top number of 120 was the goal, and one less intensive, where a top number of 140 was the goal. (Patients with diabetes and active heart disease, as well as a number of other less common health conditions, were not included, nor were those resident in a nursing home.) The question was whether the more intensive goal would reduce the rate of death, stroke, and heart attack. The short answer is yes, the group with the more intensive blood pressure goal did have fewer of these events, and it seems likely that the very fact of aiming for the more intensive goal was what did it. But the short answer is not the final answer. Rather, we should ask to whom these results apply, how big the benefit is, and whether there are any increased harms—side effects—due to aiming at stricter blood pressure control. The answers are: many people, but not everyone—not millions with kidney disease or diabetes; not those with active psychiatric illness; not those unable to tolerate many medications. The benefit? It's real but not huge—the intensive-goal group had a rate of cardiovascular events of 5.2 percent, compared to 6.8 percent in the nonintensive group (see the excellent summary of the study here: www.rxfiles.ca/rxfiles/uploads/documents/SPRINT-BP-Trial-Overview.pdf). Finally, more benefit means more side effects, ranging from effects on the kidneys to too-low blood pressure to even more serious events.

In essence, the study told us what we already knew. Increasing the intensity of blood pressure treatment can help, but it can also hurt. The risk-benefit balance is the main thing. Indeed, the main question is often not how stringently to control the blood pressure, or with what medication, but whether to use a medication.

Predicting how the medication will be tolerated ahead of time is very difficult. But conducting a trial on yourself, which in certain circles is called an N-of-1 trial, might be able to help cut through the diverse advice and disparate recommendations regarding medication treatment for hypertension.

It sounds so simple that it just might work: if you can reach a numerical target for your blood pressure without side effects that make you wonder whether you should be taking the medication, you might be doing yourself some good in a way that is sustainable over the long term.

If you reach that target with one medication and then something happens and your blood pressure increases, the instinct on the part of your doctor will be to add another medication in order to make things right or to increase the dose of the medication that you are already on. Rarely (though statistics to estimate this are difficult to come by) will a doctor suggest that you wait things out or recheck your blood pressure or perhaps examine stresses in your life that are influencing your blood pressure.

Occasionally, a blood pressure medication might stop working for you, because your body weight changes or because you have other systemic disorders that affect your blood pressure or the influence of the medication on your body—for example, kidney disease. In that case, however, your medication dose and its fittingness for you will certainly have to be reevaluated.

Most of the time, a blood pressure medicine can be taken for years. Often patients ask me how they should know whether the balance between the risk and benefit for a given medication is not right for them.

This is a good question, because that balance, in studies of medication use in populations, is generally calculated in ways that do not apply equally to every individual. Harms are calculated over groups of people, and it is impossible to predict whether they will happen to me or you.

Thus, as an individual, it might never be clear when the side effects of hypertension medicine might appear or what to do about them. This is why I would recommend a two-pronged strategy: careful monitoring of symptoms *with* the recognition that, in most cases, discontinuing blood pressure medication for a few days will not be the end of the world, presuming you have been on the medicine for some time, a few months or more.

This might sound like obvious advice, and perhaps it is, but I think many people are afraid to tell their doctors the truth about their blood pressure medicines and what taking those medicines is like for them. For example, whenever Mr. D comes to see his doctor (me), he faithfully reports that he is taking all of his medications regularly. And when I ask him, in a very open-ended way, to tell me about his blood pressure medications, he always tells me that although he did not take his blood pressure medication regularly in the past few days, he will definitely start taking them again.

What reason underlies this instinct? I think Mr. D is under the impression, which this chapter has taken pains to try and dismantle, that anti-hypertensive medications *must* be taken, day in and day out, for a lifetime and to do otherwise is to risk heart disease, kidney disease, and stroke. But there are certain circumstances in which people can take a break from them: if they cannot tolerate the medicines due to side effects, for instance, or if the pressures of life just don't allow it.

Not everyone experiences blood pressure medications the same way, and not everyone will understand the risks and benefits similarly. Not everyone will place the same pluses and minuses on the scale. To some, having to take a daily medication would be an intolerable inconvenience or just impossible given the multiple pressures of life; to others, preventing heart disease might be worth any amount of medication.

But prioritizing the pluses and minuses of a given method of treating high blood pressure requires a clear definition of those risks and benefits. For any given person—for you or me—it is impossible to predict them.

We return to an individual-centered notion of medicine. If you are diagnosed with high blood pressure and you, like Mr. D, are hemmed in by stress at work and untreated mental health issues, or if you are part of the many who are disadvantaged in our society, then it is your choice whether to decide to treat high blood pressure by medical means (e.g., medication, exercise, stress reduction) or to somehow change the social or economic situation you are in. Whatever your choice, and whatever the abilities you have to take either route, it is not your fault, and there is no "must" about it.

6

DIABETES

Sailing on the Uncertain A I C

Mr. L is a Latino man in his fifties. About ten years ago he had a lung transplant, and a few years after that, due to cancer, he had his entire colon removed. He has a large hernia in his abdomen. On top of all that, he has diabetes.

"Sometimes," he told me, "I don't really have interest in taking care of my diabetes. It is just too much."

He feels depressed a lot and doesn't eat more than a couple of times a day. He takes insulin twice daily.

I asked him at his last visit how he thinks his diabetes is being controlled and he said, "Not that badly, actually," but he couldn't tell me how high his sugar was at home, and the more we talked, the more apparent it was that his sugar was really high at home. Really high, for those who know diabetes, means in the 200s or 300s (milligrams per deciliter) during the day.

Those reading this who know about diabetes will nod their head. They know what these numbers mean and what the targets are. They have found a way to live with diabetes. They know that living with a disease does not necessarily mean just conforming to the advice of their doctor—it means making all the information and the advice work for them.

How do we bridge the doctors' advice, full of numbers, directions, and scientific studies, with the life that we have to live? How do we figure out how to treat diabetes our own way, while also realizing that we are not the experts in how "best" to live with diabetes? In other words, how do we make the scientific lingo of medicine work for us as ordinary individuals with diabetes?

I have made reference more than once in this book to a concept outlined by Annemarie Moll in *The Logic of Care*: distinguishing decision making from the process of practice—trial and error through time—that characterizes the experience of life with a disease.

Often, as patients we do not make discrete decisions in living with a disease but negotiate various pathways in order to continue the course of our life under its influence. However, sometimes a third logic does apply to existing with a medical diagnosis: not the logic of decision making (in which the voyage with diabetes, say, is viewed as a series of discrete decision points or intersections) and not the logic of care (in which life with the disease is viewed through the prism of *phronesis*—that is, a kind of moral practice) but that of advice seeking. There is a right way and a wrong way to proceed: not in the trial-and-error way of Moll's practice, yet not according to the strict definitions of the biomedical paradigm.

The fact that we need advice from an expert, though we recognize that the expert is imperfect, speaks to one of the central dilemmas of medicine today. On the one hand, we have the dictates of so-called evidence-based medicine. As we discussed in previous chapters, such evidence can be imperfect, biased, inaccurate, wrong, and, what's worse, completely without insight regarding the extent to which it departs from truth.

We have recognized that when we go to the doctor, we want to be in charge—or else be given the real alternative of actually being in charge. We want to be recognized as the ones who should set the priorities of our care. By the same token, however, our priorities are not always reachable by ourselves alone, especially in the context of illness. Medical expertise, no matter how imperfect it might be, helps determine courses of action, potential goals, outcomes, and even priorities for our lives.

Thus, in diabetes, as with other conditions, we cannot easily escape this meeting of dilemmas, the imperfect evidence base and the uncertain patient, because evidence is always imperfect and we are always somewhat uncertain.

The dilemma was expertly summarized recently by the physician-blogger Richard Lehman in his entertaining, enlightening, and curmudgeonly countercultural blog at the *British Medical Journal*:

I would just like to propose two common scenarios. A Bangladeshi woman of 34 is found to have high blood sugar and raised BP in her third pregnancy: these persist and within two years she is on six different medications including increasing doses of insulin. Her BMI is 41, she does not speak English and usually attends the practice nurse with a family member.

Secondly, a 73 year old white male was found to have a BP of 164/96 ten years ago and has been on two antihypertensive drugs since. He has also been taking metformin for 5 years and his HbA1c runs at about 8 and his BMI is 32.

Now I just want you to ask yourself: what are the absolute risks of cardiovascular disease, blindness, amputation and renal failure and the absolute benefits of each element of management (including surgery and lifestyle change) in either of these people? How are you going to communicate them and achieve the goals that your patient would most like? Do these people in fact have anything in common except a pair of labels ("hypertension" and "type 2 diabetes")? What real-life questions would you like to see answered by new forms of what we now call meta-analysis?[1]

Lehman is speaking to doctors here. We can put it in normal-person terms like this: According to the biomedical model of disease treatment, in which we have problems that medicine can correct, the reason to participate in diabetes treatment is to reduce the frequency of certain outcomes. We would take medicine or change our diet or do something else in order to keep us from developing future complications that we would like to avoid.

Every part of the above assumption can be determined by randomized trials, scientific studies that are considered the gold standard. However, at the very same time, each of the above assumptions can be questioned by any individual.

"Participating in diabetes treatment can lead to improvement in outcomes." Outcomes run the gamut. It would be one thing if we were sure that taking a particular group of treatments for diabetes would increase the number of high-quality years we have left to live. For instance, if we were told that taking insulin would increase our survival, decreasing the number of heart attacks among those with diabetes, that might make matters simpler for many of us. Unfortunately, it is not so simple. In general, treatment for diabetes *can* favorably impact (decrease) rates of heart attack, stroke, and other blood-vessel-related diseases, things that people would like to avoid, but this does not necessarily mean that we will live longer if we take these medications.

There are other clear benefits for diabetes treatments: decreased rates of eye disease and problems with the peripheral nerves, so-called microvascular disease.[2] For some of us, these outcomes might matter just as much as heart disease or stroke.

But for each of these multifarious outcomes, we need to balance the benefit of the particular medication regimen with the potential downsides for us. No matter how detailed the potential list of benefits, we can be sure of one thing: for us as individuals, the medications will have a very specific effect that they will not have for anyone else.

There is a recently arisen but already very broad area of research that is meant to apply the specific findings of scientific trials to the goals that matter to ordinary patients. Such patient-centered research has given rise to an entirely federally funded institute of its own: the Patient-Centered Outcomes Research Institute (PCORI). The enterprise is meant to help researchers and clinicians focus on the results that matter to us, ordinary people.

This attempt is wholly salutary. However, even if PCORI's attempt to pursue such research is wholly successful, it still won't answer the needs of the patient whose story I started telling above. If Mr. L's greatest priority is to be able to reduce his weight so that his painful abdominal hernia can be corrected, no study in the world will be able to balance the various effects of different diabetes medications, with their potential harms, for the timescale that matters to him—that is, in the years in which getting that abdominal surgery might be a possibility.

One would have to factor into the decision not just the benefits and harms for each potential course of action but also the likelihood that those actions would lead to the outcome that mattered to Mr. L the most. And the benefits, harms, and likelihoods would have to include the immediate risks and benefits immediately attributable to medications (such as are listed in the results of randomized controlled trials that are used to determine the effectiveness of medications and secure their government approval), as well as the harms and benefits attributable to a given course of treatment down the line.

Even though the logic of decision making isn't, to agree with Moll, the only right outlook on the complicated business of getting the right health care for us, sometimes we do need to focus on decisions. It's just that the decisions involve consequences distant from the decision itself. And in between the medication (or whatever treatment option we pick) and the downstream consequences, life can happen, in all its manifold twists and turns, rendering irrelevant the complicated balancing we have performed when thinking about options or discussing them with a doctor or loved one.

What can we do about this as patients with diabetes or as those taking care of someone with diabetes? The problem is not just that the treatment options for diabetes involve harms and that tracking the blood sugars, changing diet, and undertaking regular exercise—all potential routes to treat the disease—are difficult. These might apply to any medical condition. It is that the balance of benefits and harms most relevant to us for any possible combination of treatments is not likely to be fully recognized by the health care worker we are talking to, and, as a result, we are likely to be put into any one of a number of boxes. These boxes are the confining choices appropriate to an algorithm, and many doctors and patients refer to such an algorithm even when the evidence does not support them. To take one example, it has for some years been accepted by many practitioners that those with diabetes need to have their care tailored to a particular value of the so-called glycohemoglobins (hemoglobin A1C) lab values, which show what the value of blood sugar has been over the past few months.

Make no mistake, such lab tests have been of incredible value in the diagnosis and treatment of diabetes. They are more accurate in diagnosing the disease than a simple blood-sugar finger stick, and they help track the treatment of the disease. However, as is so often the case in advanced medicine, the presence of a test does not necessarily, uncomplicatedly lead to better care.

The problem, as far as the ordinary person is concerned, is that both a low hemoglobin A1C value and a high A1C can be associated with benefits or harms. A hemoglobin A1C of less than 7 can be associated with a range of harms in populations, including increased mortality.[3] The harms are particularly relevant in older people.[4] Further, if for some reason you have gotten this test and, with a value greater than 6.5 percent, you are told that this confers upon you a diagnosis of diabetes, you should be careful when accepting the diagnosis. A diagnosis can be therapeutic and can empower you, but it can also set upon you the demons of overuse. The first treatment for your diabetes might very well be the thing you were planning on doing anyway: weight loss, a healthier diet, and regular exercise.

People and lives are more complicated than numbers, as we have learned time and time again. Someone in these age groups, perhaps you or someone you know, might choose to identify a goal for sugar control that does not conform to these numbers simply because in many cases the studies of diabetics do not include geriatric populations and likely are not entirely generalizable to your circumstance.

Many will say that, lacking better evidence, it makes sense to go along with the recommendations of these organizations, well-respected groups of doctors and patients such as the American Diabetes Association, or groups that help summarize the medical evidence, such as the U.S. Preventive Services Task Force. This is a reasonable approach if it seems right to you. What I am trying to point out here is that seeing these numbers as an our-way-or-the-highway life-or-death decision is unrealistic and does not accord with the imperfections of the science or the complications and uniqueness of you as an individual.

For those starting out on the journey of a life with type 2 diabetes (type 1 is a different matter, which we will not discuss here) or for those dissatisfied with their current direction of care, there are potential routes to self-treatment, with the help of a doctor, that can reduce the risk of macrovascular disease (heart attack, stroke) and microvascular complications (nerve damage and eye disease).

This is one of the few diseases in which present-day technology, when made generally available, can lead to improvements in control that might, in turn, lead to real advances in patient-related outcomes.

Insulin pumps can, if made available to populations, help smooth the curves of insulin supply, which cause people great expenditures of time and effort.

Apart from these methods, however, and if these technologies are not available to you, take a route to diabetes treatment that feels right to you. You do not need to start on a medication as your first route to treatment if you would rather not, even if your doctor is recommending otherwise. This is because many people with diabetes are perfectly able to control their diet and increase their exercise, both things that can bring their blood sugar down.

I hear some of the other doctors squawking out there in the medical world, however. "If the patient does not start a medication right away, they are putting themselves at risk for the effects of high blood sugar!" Perhaps. But any one of us might weigh our preference for staying off medications as long as possible more strongly than the theoretical numerical benefit of keeping our blood sugar in a particular range. That is, the hemoglobin A1C might not matter to us if we have diabetes, even if it is established through scientific studies that a hemoglobin A1C out of the preferred range will increase our risk for heart disease or stroke.

That doesn't mean we want to get those diseases, just that some of us want to avoid medication for as long as possible.

I have a patient, Ms. V, who has had diabetes as long as I have been treating her. And for as long as I have known her, she has not wanted to take insulin. She knows all about insulin because her sister used it for years. Her hemoglobin A1C has defiantly stayed in the region of 8–10. Sometimes up, sometimes down, never controlled according to the numerical algorithms that sometimes we need to look beyond.

At every visit, because I want to be a doctor who follows the rules, I ask her whether she will consider taking insulin in order to better control her diabetes. "I don't want to be on insulin," she says. "I am scared of needles."

On her most recent visit, I got sick of playing the nice guy and put it out there: "If we better control your blood sugar, we can reduce your risk of heart disease or stroke or the other things that diabetes may cause. We can protect your eyes and kidneys and feet."

She looked at me. "Is that true?"

I nodded my head.

"So you can guarantee me that if I take insulin, I won't get a heart attack or stroke, my kidneys, eyes, and feet will be protected?"

I prevaricated. "Ah," she said, "I could take insulin and have these things happen to me anyway."

Although I tried to point out that her risk would be less, her fear of needles won out that day.

This difference between what is predicted for populations and what individuals decide is particularly acute in diabetes because it is often described as an epidemic. Indeed, the incidence of diabetes is increasing. And according to one conception of health promotion, a problem widespread in populations needs to be confronted with an intervention on a population scale. There is a lot of breast cancer, so we need to promote mammograms; there is a lot of smoking, so we should tell people to stop.

By the same token, we should test for diabetes and control it for as many people as we can.

As individuals, we do need to care about the care of populations, because, as I have pointed out elsewhere in this book, inequalities in the way health services are available from one group to another can affect the health of each of us. But this doesn't mean that each of us should behave according to guidelines developed for populations. Even if a certain collection of recommendations might decrease our risk of heart attack or stroke or of disease affecting the eyes, kidneys, or limbs, we can still say no to them.

WHAT GOAL SHOULD WE ADOPT FOR OURSELVES?

Is there a way to use the impressive tools developed for physicians and use them for our own individual care (ideally, with the help of a primary care provider we know and trust)? If the hemoglobin A1C goals do not work the same way for every individual, is there a way we can modify these goals for each person?

The problem is that the data can't be sliced thin enough in the way research is done now. The American Diabetes Association recommends that older adults have higher hemoglobin A1C goals (i.e., that more hyperglycemia be allowed for older individuals), but millions of people fall into the category of "older individuals." And while categories do very well for classifying risk for the purposes of a study, each one of us has a different way of balancing what is important for us.

Will there come a time when I know what hemoglobin A1C number is right for me personally—that is, whether I should aim for 6.5 percent, 7 percent, or 8 percent?

We can retain scientific hopes, perhaps not fantasies, that might come true in the service of personalizing our risks. There is much relevant scientific research going on in this field—how to specify the individual risk of disease. The science of epidemiology has been progressing in this direction for decades already. The landmark Framingham study helped establish for the first time the risk factors that would make it more likely for a person to develop heart disease, and similar risk factors have been analyzed in the case of diabetes. Science has advanced since that time, and now the risk-factor discussion has less to do with behaviors (e.g., smoking) or levels of cholesterol and blood pressure; the emphasis is now placed ever more on genetic risk.

The promise of precision medicine has been ever more amplified in the media and the press releases of top-flight medical centers and research institutions. *Precision medicine* means using the genetic information particular to a given individual in order to tailor their treatment to them "precisely." The prospect of treating each person according to their individual characteristics is exciting, thrilling even. Imagine that you could put your individual, personal self in the hands of the health care system, knowing that science had figured out how to apply medical treatment to your particular combination of genes and proteins!

Given the experience of living with diabetes that we have explored in this chapter, the promise of precision medicine is even more attractive. Rather than figuring out how to get your sugar into the box of particular values (80–130 mg/dL when fasting) or trying to improve your hemoglobin A1C without knowing whether a particular numerical range is right for you, you can look to your genes to provide information about which medications might be best for you personally.

Precision medicine, in other words, is just another kind of risk stratification but is based on genetic research—at least in the version popularized by the White House in its recent initiative.[5]

This is disappointing, because precision medicine, when used in other diseases, at its best has achieved . . . not so much. Of the ballyhooed benefits supposed to redound to us from the massive initiative to sequence the human genome, perhaps only a medication for cystic fibrosis can be confidently pointed to.[6]

There are two responses to the overblown promises made for precision medicine. One is to expand the definition of the concept. Precision medicine comes from the world of clinical research, which focuses on the individual to the exclusion of public health.[7] That is, precision medicine is mistaken because it does not consider the health needs of populations.

This objection is well intentioned but misses the mark. As I have pointed out, part of the problem with today's clinical care as it relates to those with diabetes is that principles of public health do not necessarily apply to the care of the individual. Universal screening does not aim at your own individual concerns, and the hemoglobin A1C guidelines do not take into account your unique priorities.

The other way to approach precision medicine from a realistically feasible point of view is to understand that identifying individual factors extends far beyond molecules. Genes and proteins are important but do not specify behaviors, outcomes, or risks. We are not our molecules but fully individual beings in a matrix of family, friends, neighborhoods, and society. This is not public health, because we cannot on a large, population scale intervene in neighborhood health factors, but learning about the myriad of influences that impinge on the life of each of us. Many researchers are starting to realize this.[8]

A different way to make precision medicine feasible has to do with Bayesian statistics, an approach to statistics that involves modifying our previously held estimates of the likelihood that given states of affairs are true. Using such statistics, which have been around for a long time, can help researchers understand whether different categories of patients are helped by the treatments evaluated in clinical studies—even if these are not the categories that the study was originally designed to address.[9]

EVEN CORRECTED, PRECISION MEDICINE IS NOT ENOUGH TO "CURE" DIABETES

The claims that precision medicine can cure diabetes can be forgiven as excited exaggerations. But the idea that the above corrections can make precision medicine a significant advance in the treatment of diabetes is also an exaggeration.

How many chronic diseases can we really have been said to "cure"? Perhaps we have cured the hepatitis C virus through a remarkable, though hugely expensive, new medication.[10] However, the cost of the medication itself, and the burden it places on society, raises this question: What does a cure mean when it is not equally available for all?

Another cure that we can say was accomplished is the discovery and treatment of *Helicobacter pylori* as the causative organism of ulcers.[11] Treatment of this organism with antibiotics leads to a significantly improved rate of ulcer treatment. Yet compliance with this treatment is difficult, given the multiple number of medications that compose it, taken over a number of weeks. Further, antibiotic resistance is a significant issue with the treatment of *H. pylori*, and treatment must be modified to acknowledge this fact, an effort that is pursued infrequently.[12]

Hepatitis C and *Helicobacter pylori* are both infectious agents—one a virus, one a bacteria—so it is reasonable to speak of a possible "cure" for them. However, most chronic diseases are the result of a confluence of factors, such that it doesn't make much sense to speak of a single cure. This is also true of diabetes: the disease is not just due to a lack of insulin but also (in type 2 diabetes) to a decreased sensitivity to its action; not just diet but also physical activity, home, and work; not just sugar, when you come down to it, but also other risk factors for heart disease.

A cure for diabetes would need to bring all these factors, somehow, into synergy and fix each of them. Appreciating the manifold factors that impact diabetes is enough to see how ridiculous is the claim for a cure through precision medicine.

What should we aim at, then, as a society, as researchers, as clinicians, as people with diabetes? We cannot live without hope, without something to aim at just over the next obstacle. I have already described some directions that many have taken—to my mind, mistakenly or, rather, if not wrongheaded in themselves, lacking when pursued as a global strategy for diabetes—the public health strategy, in which population criteria should define the care of an individual; precision medicine, according to which the genes of an individual, or, in a corrected version, her or his social environment as well, should dictate the treatment.

Our hope and ambition should be this: if we have diabetes, that we can pursue the best care possible according to our individual preferences; and if we are taking care of someone with diabetes, that we do not become trapped by population measures when the person's preferences dictate something different.

7

ARTHRITIS

What's Bred in the Bone

Ms. B came into my office with her walker, a half-smile, and a groan. She was born in France. Living in Baltimore since 1956 (down the street from where I live, with a carefully tended garden), she still bears a trace of a French accent and used to regale me with tales of her voyages from one farm to another on returning to her own neck of the woods in the South of France. On those occasions, I was happy to hear about her indulgences in rich pastries and fine wines, impressed that she had managed to clamber up and down medieval stone paths on the journey to this or that old church.

But that was some time ago. For the past couple of years, she has had pain in her left knee and leg that she can't bear, and she has come in to see me about it quite frequently, more or less every month. Every visit has been heralded by the familiar groan: "Oh, Dr. Berger, my knee hurts so much."

Sometimes she comes in with her two sons, who sit and listen (usually in good humor, sometimes with a trifle impatience) to the nth recounting of her tale of woe. Sometimes she is alone. But the pain is her predominant preoccupation, at least when she is in the office with me.

"What can we do about my pain, Dr. Berger?"

The first step, according to the biomedical paradigm (diagnose, then treat), is often to figure out the cause. And as is often the case, her pain had not one but many causes. Some of it was due to overstretch in her lower leg—or, to put it another way, Achilles tendon problems. Some of it likely has to do with the nerve problems and associated pain (neuropathy) caused by her diabetes. Her depression (her mood has worsened over the last few years) and sleeping problems unfortunately do not make any of this easier.

But the cause that looms largest among all of the others is arthritis. She always mentions her arthritis during every visit. "What are we going to do about my arthritis?" And lest I think this is something she only brings up during her visits with me, her sons tell me that she also mentions her arthritis frequently at home, when cataloging her pain complaints.

As her doctor, one thing that fascinates me is the predominance of arthritis among the problems that receive her attention. I don't doubt for a minute that pain is one of the most fatiguing and life-changing symptoms. Thus, it is not surprising that she talks about her pain the most. What I find remarkable is the extent to which arthritis as a cause of this pain occupies pride of place in her pain narrative. The tendinitis is something we discuss over and over again, and we lavish attention on the diabetes, but we always return to the arthritis as a leitmotif.

I can't prove it, and I am not sure that Ms. B would appreciate the question if I asked, but I think that she sees arthritis as more important than her other ailments because there is a potential solution that can fix it: knee replacement surgery. She focuses on her arthritis because she thinks it can be solved.

I am exaggerating somewhat, because Ms. B has not always been requesting knee surgery. We have known each other for years, and as her symptoms have become worse, and as her mobility correspondingly decreases, she has only started mentioning knee replacement with increasing frequency in the past year. That is because her pain is getting worse but also because knee replacement is seen as "the only cure" to arthritis.

There is a grain of truth in this. If osteoarthritis in its final stages (known colloquially as "bone on bone") is a dysfunction of the joint itself, then replacing the joint is a true advance, replacing the broken by the fixed. This is a byproduct of the biomedical paradigm: figuring out what in the body is broken, then going and fixing it. Other examples of this paradigm abound in everyday practice. Heart vessels, when blocked, cause decreased blood supply to the heart tissue, pain, and then tissue death, so we should relieve that blockage. Depression involves an imbalance in the brain's neurochemistry, so we should redress that balance. Diabetes is due to a deficiency of insulin or a decreased sensitivity to that protein in the body, so we should give the body more or make it more sensitive.

But all of the examples in the above paragraph are incomplete or misleading. Heart tissue, when not in the throes of a heart attack, can function with incomplete blockages of the vessel—thus, it is not clear that intervening on such blockages (putting in a stent to make sure that blockages do not happen, engaging in surgery to remove blockages) is better than making sure that other, less invasive treatments are being tailored to our needs.[1] As I discuss elsewhere, depression medications are not the only way to treat depression, and therapy sometimes does just as well. Diabetes, similarly, can be treated in a host of ways other than with insulin.

Thus, in short, the biomedical assumption that knowing what is broken will tell us how to fix it is not always justified. And this leads to important consequences in how we should understand how to treat our bodies when they are broken.

Back to Ms. B. In short, she kept mentioning the pain in her knee because she had it. She was sure it was due to arthritis (a reasonable assumption, though, as we pointed out above, the pain could be worsened by other factors as well). And because it was due to arthritis, it should be fixed.

But should it be?

The open secret of any surgery is also the reason why good surgeons are good: the best ones carefully choose, based on their experience and the scientific literature (and perhaps not on anything definable at all), which patients will do best with a given surgery. Even as an acolyte of peer-reviewed, evidence-based medicine, the judgment of surgeons makes a lot of sense to me. They are ready to operate on . . . who they think is appropriate to be operated on, the sort of person they think the procedure will help.

Those of us whom surgeons would not even let across the threshold of their operating room don't make it into randomized trials of surgery, so the results of those studies cannot be generalized to the many of us who have significant disease or other reasons that make surgery difficult or potentially ineffective. When it comes to bridging the gap between evidence-based medicine and patient preference, in the case of surgery, we are even more lost than in other health care questions; for the sickest of us (if we are taking fifteen medications or aren't that active to start with or have active psychiatric disease), the trials might not apply, and we only have the expert's say-so to go on.

Ms. B was bitterly disappointed when the surgeon refused to replace her knee about a month ago. Her blood sugar was too high. As her primary care doctor, I did not refuse to refer her to the surgeon in the first place, but I was very skeptical that the knee replacement would work at all. I had no joy, nevertheless, that the surgeon sent her right back to me without laying hands on her. I wanted her to get her pain treated. I wanted her to have the curative procedure.

We met after the surgeon made that decision; she was distraught. She has a history of depression, not a Gallic personality trait but a clinical condition that we have previously discussed treating, but she told me it was worse. "Because the doctor said he wouldn't do the knee operation."

The barrier to Ms. B getting her knee replaced is, of course, her diabetes. But also in the way, for her, is insulin: the thing I keep recommending to her and the route she does not want to take. She is "scared of needles," she has told me honestly several times. She is not sure her diabetes is as badly controlled as all that. And even though she nods in seeming agreement when I explain how her high blood sugar affects the chance of complications from surgery and why the surgeon might, for that reason, refuse to perform the operation, I am not sure that she has internalized this barrier in a way that she understands.

If you were in Ms. B's position, what would you do? Let's give you some options to help you work through what your preferences might be and to prepare you for a situation in which you might be faced with this sort of decision.

1. You would want your knee to be replaced and would therefore at least be willing to give insulin a try so that the surgeon might feel comfortable about the joint replacement. Whatever worry you had about insulin would pale in comparison to the desire you had to get your knee fixed since the pain had been bothering you for some time.

2. You would want your knee to get replaced, but you would still be worried about starting insulin. You have heard things about its side effects, and you are on no account ready to start giving yourself

injections. Since the time you were diagnosed with diabetes, you have been sure that you will not be able to tolerate injections. So you will add another diabetes medication if your doctor advises it.

3. You are really worried about changing your medication regimen for your diabetes. Actually, though your doctor says it is out of control, you feel very well and are looking forward to going on vacation. You are not sure your diabetes is as poorly controlled as all that.

4. You don't know what to do but would love it if the surgeon were to replace your knee as he said he might.

These alternatives do not include the idea that the knee replacement might not help as much as you have been hoping. This is the alternative I have been bringing up with Ms. B time and again as her physician and the one that has seemed to have difficulty gaining purchase with her.

Ms. B is not alone in her optimistic expectations about the result of knee surgery. In a recent study published in the journal *Health Expectations*,[2] a group of internal medicine physicians, public health scientists, and orthopedists surveyed 236 patients at a single orthopedics center in Texas before their total knee replacement, asking them how long they thought it would take them to recover, resume normal activities, and be free from pain. Sixty-five percent expected to be functionally recovered—back to the activities they used to do—after three months. Eighty percent of people surveyed expected that three months after the survey they would be able to perform at least eight of ten common activities (e.g., putting on socks, driving, walking without a cane, etc.). Most remarkably, 62 percent believed they would walk one block without a cane at six weeks, not an unrealistic expectation but certainly on the optimistic side of the spectrum.

How does this compare to the experiences of people who have undergone such surgery? Unsurprisingly, the match is not exact. In short, if you were to say that knee replacement gets rid of the problem by substituting a new, perfectly functioning joint for an old, painful joint, you would be exaggerating the case. Two years ago, Andrew David Beswick and others, in the journal *BMJ Open*, reviewed studies that estimated the proportion of patients who had hip or knee replacement, and they found that the proportion of those with an unfavorable outcome after knee replacement was about 34 percent. That is, one in three patients who had their knee replaced were not satisfied with the pain outcome after surgery.[3] (Interestingly enough, the proportion of patients who were dissatisfied with hip surgery was found to be somewhat lower, perhaps because their expectations before surgery were limited.)

That last research finding helps us understand such a situation in general but does not help in understanding how I should help Ms. B navigate among the options listed above. She has already made her decision: she wants to have the knee replaced. If I were to tell her about the chance she might be dissatisfied after the operation, would it influence her decisions? And would it be the right thing to do?

The answer to this question gets at the difference between us deciding what we want and us, together with doctors, deciding what is right for us.

If we think the priority is to make Ms. B the driver of her own health care and help her make her own decisions, then her goal should be to have that knee replacement, regardless of the chance that she might have some nonsignificant risk of dissatisfaction after the procedure. Call this the "knee replacement come hell or high water" option. Put yourself in Ms. B's place, and it might be easier to see how this option could be the one she chooses.

If the goal is to pursue shared decision making, where doctor and patient work together in a partnership, then she might very well decide, after listening to the doctor's advice, that the knee replacement is really not for her—it might not make her feel better after all, and the complications of the diabetes might make it difficult to ensure a completely smooth and complication-free outcome.

However, Ms. B is the type of person who is not used to talking explicitly about the ways in which she would like her decision to be made. Like most of us in the health care system, *decision making* and *autonomy* are terms used by researchers, not by people in the course of their ordinary consideration of alternatives. I do not know if that is because Ms. B prefers for the decisions to be made by her doctor (there is certainly a proportion of patients who feel that way) or because she thinks the decision has already been made by her surgeon or because she has not arrived at the understanding that she can actually express her preferences—in short, she might think that what she wants matters but is happy to see it dictated from the outside, by the doctor-as-expert.

If the expectations of Ms. B will not necessarily match the outcomes of her knee surgery, but she wants the surgery and her diabetes is getting in the way, what can we do about it? On the one hand, what will happen in this particular situation might not really depend on my role as Ms. B's doctor. I have raised my concerns with her multiple times and tried to get her to understand that I do not think that her knee replacement will help her get rid of her pain. I don't think she as an individual is going to change her decision, and, while I am not sure her symptoms will be cured by a knee replacement as she is hoping, the knee replacement as a procedure is still in the spectrum of practice, such that I feel comfortable helping her make it happen. There are things that "doctors do" for people with knee arthritis and severe pain, and knee replacement is one of them.

How can we make it easier for people to make decisions about their arthritis?

We should realize that expectations are not necessarily aligned with the reality of what happens after such procedures.

Do we remove knee replacement from the armamentarium or try and encourage people to have it done less often? Should we regulate it so that it is done at lower levels? Or provide incentives so that surgeons will improve their process based on outcomes that matter to ordinary people, such that there is less residual pain after the procedure?

Perhaps these options are all possible. But I have a feeling, perhaps just a hunch, that a culture change is needed to modify how we look at knee replacement (and perhaps all joint replacement). The realization needs to percolate through the world of patients with knee problems (starting with you reading this book, perhaps) that knee surgery is not all that it is cracked up to be.

Are there previous instances of surgeries that have risen in popularity and then readjusted to lower levels? I don't think there are, at least not in the contemporary United States. Actually, the examples of surgical procedures that come to mind are all those that are becoming more frequent or at least not decreasing in frequency, despite dubious evidence of their effectiveness. Or, put another way, these procedures are happening more often than necessary.

One example is an appendectomy for appendicitis. One study found that the rate of diagnosis of appendicitis (and resulting appendectomy) has increased from 7.62 to 9.38 per 10,000 patients between 1993 and 2008,[4] despite active controversy in the literature about the necessity for these appendectomies. Perhaps (as in Europe) they should be treated with antibiotics first.[5] Take another example: cesarean sections have increased as a percentage of all births from 20.7 percent in 1996 to 31.1 percent in 2006. Cesarean rates increased for women of all ages, race/ethnic groups, and gestational ages and in all states. [6]

Perhaps the intervention should be the same sort that is being implemented in other areas of the health care system: payment shifts to decrease the incentive that leads doctors and other health care professionals to behave as if more is always better. It stands to reason that if doctors are paid for the services they do, with "services" including anything countable, like a procedure or a hospitalization or a test, then they will do more of them. (Granted, the truth is somewhat more complicated, since many physicians are not directly reimbursed more based on the number of procedures they do, but the phenomenon has become so widespread that there are now multiple economic incentives baked into the system, far outstripping mere salary.) [7]

The trick is to find ways to reimburse doctors and others fairly for the work they do while not incentivizing them to do procedures for their own sake.

In the case of Ms. B, even if she is bound and determined to get her knee surgery, perhaps there would be mechanisms in place to ensure that she understands, or at least can informedly refuse, the potential likelihood that the knee surgery might not reduce her symptoms significantly.

This might require improved doctor-patient communication, not in the sense of a one-way recitation of risks and benefits, which passes for communication in some quarters, but (as I detail in *Talking to Your Doctor*) a real conversation between two people with a stake in their health-promoting relationship. [8]

This means, as in any relationship, that Ms. B and I could both do better. I can do better by her in presenting a wider range of options to help her knee pain and thinking about how to deemphasize surgery while still giving realistic estimates about what would happen were she to go through with it.

My job in this improved relationship would not be to say no to the Ms. Bs of the world who come expecting knee replacement surgery but to place their expectations about knee replacement surgery in the context of what people actually undergo and how they feel afterward—perhaps through arranged interviews with people like them or by providing narratives (e.g., on video) from those who have had such surgery. In the same way that stories about someone's colostomy (an artificial outlet created for the exit of bowel contents after some or much of the bowel is excised for other medical reasons) can help people feel more confident about choosing that route,[9] stories about the experiences of people who have had total knee replacement might make expectations more realistic.

If I could do better for Ms. B, then she could do better for herself. I do not mean here that her arthritis symptoms are, by any stretch of the imagination, her fault but that she could expect more from me while still honoring her own preferences.

She could ask me to map out the possibilities for the development of her knee arthritis. How would her symptoms look in the future? What would her functional ability look like with medication? With different types of medication compared to each other? Would each of them improve, have little effect on, or potentially worsen her general state: the number of feet she could walk unassisted, the pain she would have, the money she would spend on medications?

What would physical therapy do for her symptoms (her pain) and/or her activity?

And, finally, what would surgery do? What could she expect from the procedure, how much time would it take her to recuperate, and how would this compare to the nonsurgical options?

Would she be right to expect this exhaustive option-mapping from me? Haven't I been saying time and again in this book that this is precisely what can't be predicted? Aren't I of the opinion that any such estimates are unreliable because they try to make applicable to the individual what we only know from population-based studies?

True enough, but Ms. B and her family are looking to me for answers. If we lived in a different health care environment—one in which incentives did not aim toward procedures but toward providing the best care for a given condition, one in which every patient was expected to be provided with the means to make decisions for themselves, and one in which our expectations were not for cures but for ameliorating treatments—then perhaps she would not have to come to me to "tell her what to do" (even though that is something I am reluctant to do, as a matter of fact). If health care were more decentralized, if physical therapy could be obtained without a doctor's prescription, if a wider range of pain medications was more widely available, and if physical activity were more a part of life and more easily available, even for those in her age group and relative lack of mobility, all these things would make my job less essential.

However, arthritis, like life itself and our health care system, is a byproduct of imperfection. Joints wear out, and there is nothing much we can do about them that is curative and perfect and without harms or imperfections. Put another way, if things were different, there would not be joint degeneration at all. But there is, and joint replacement, though a valuable option, is just one among many, and there is nothing we can point Ms. B toward without qualms and complications and qualifications.

Tending away from the curative and toward the ameliorative is appropriate for arthritis, just as with the other conditions in this book, but for slightly different reasons and appropriate to the particular circumstances of Ms. B as well. Osteoarthritis can be improved through mobility—that is, either home exercises or "aerobic" walking (walking strenuous enough to require increased breathing and heart rate).[10] If we have arthritis, we need to understand this suggestion in the proper context. It is by no means equivalent to saying, "Well, if you just got up and *got moving*, all your arthritis symptoms would go away"—this is cruel, untrue, and unhelpful. But engaging in the activities of life, to the extent that one's pain allows, can in itself be a way to draw a circle around symptoms and to emphasize amelioration rather than cure.

There is still much we do not know about arthritis, of course—but that's not really the point. A cure for everyone who suffers from this disease is not forthcoming, nor should that be what we, as those with arthritis, look forward to. We need to find the best treatments for us among the options available, with the support of someone who can walk through them with us. In the end, amelioration should be our goal, as people with the disease, as caregivers, and as practitioners. Or, if "cure" is to be the direction that we tend to, we should in the same breath openly acknowledge the risks and downsides that come with that approach.

8

SURGERY

To Be Operated On or Not—and with Whom?

I am not a surgeon. That is obvious to anyone who knows me: I am legally blind and not particularly coordinated (though I am able to physically examine patients with expertise, by dint of years of practice). I remember when I was a medical student on my surgery rotation and an experienced surgeon, wishing to entertain me (I was obviously bored, about to fall over, several hours into some sort of long, complicated operation), gave an excited little shout: "That's the aorta!"

I saw the fat sausage that controls a hugely significant blood flow, and my boredom immediately turned to terror. "Put it away!" I didn't want to break it or have anything happen to it.

My specialty, internal medicine, is naturally paired with a healthy respect for surgeons. Internists and surgeons see different sorts of patients, which influences how we understand the risks and benefits of surgery. Surgeons see the people for whom operations work, or at least for whom a surgical procedure can be considered. Internal medicine doctors, by and large, see those people who don't need surgery, who get better without it, and who don't really want to have surgery. (Those who are more acutely ill often tend to be seen in emergency departments or urgent care centers, finding their way to surgeons.) Both of us, internists and surgeons, see those who undergo harms from surgery.

Since I don't do the operations myself (nor would you want me to), this chapter is not about how to do surgery but about how to decide whether surgery is the right thing for you. The decision of whether to have surgery is both similar to and quite unlike the other health conditions I discuss in this book. It is similar because it involves a decision: whether to have a surgery is something like whether to use insulin for diabetes, which treatment for hypertension to adopt (or any at all), whether to pursue chemotherapy for cancer, which might extend survival by some amount in return for a collection of harms and side effects.

The same ingredients go into any decision. Theoretically (e.g., in the large economic literature on decision making), they involve not just strictly numerical judgments on risks and benefits but also behavioral—that is to say, psychological—judgments, made famous in the Nobel Prize–winning work of Amos Tversky and Daniel Kahneman[1] and in medicine by the work of Peter Ubel, among others.[2] In essence, when we have to make a medical decision, we do not consider merely the numerical estimates of what benefits might accrue to us from each option, balancing them with the harms that might occur. Rather, we approach any decision with the psychological techniques that we have evolved (or, depending on how you understand their development, which have developed in the context of societal pressures) to aid us in dealing with incomplete information that we deal with irrationally.

But surgical decisions are different from other decisions in important ways: the options are reduced. The context is no longer about what the problem is, how we got here, what to do about it, and how to move forward, but rather narrowed to "Should one have surgery?"

The fact of the matter is, though we would like for all options to be revealed to us at every point, so we could get a broad sense of what to do from all directions, we often receive a very restricted view of the options because everyone we are talking to has their biases. It is unlikely that a doctor will tell us to do nothing about our hypertension, otherwise she would not have diagnosed it. People go to gastroenterologists, more or less, so that their gastroenterologic tract can be looked at from the inside. And so on. Similarly, surgeons are visited so that surgery can be seriously considered. This is not controversial.

The first direction we should follow when visiting a surgeon is to hurry up and wait a minute. Unless we or our loved ones are, God forbid, in extremis or acutely ill—for example, we are bleeding at a life-threatening rate or have a growing mass somewhere—there is no reason not to wait and deliberate about the place of surgery among our options. Many is the time that someone has asked me, as their doctor, if they "should" or "must" have knee replacement surgery. Knee surgery can help symptoms, but except for cases of trauma, in my experience, there is no "must" about it. It is a weighing of benefits and harms.

Deciding whether to have surgery should take into account the same factors we have discussed in other chapters: the benefits (relief of symptoms, most commonly, at least for elective procedures such as spinal surgery or knee replacement) versus the harms. What makes deciding about surgery different is that we should also figure out the way, place, person, and time to have it done.

If you are considering surgery, you might likely have little choice about where to have it done. This choice might be limited by your insurance plan or geographical convenience. If an academic medical center is convenient to you, you might be able to choose among a number of surgeons with the help of online aids such as Physician Compare or Hospital Compare, but the numbers these lists show might not always be relevant to the outcomes you care about. Similarly, there is cost information available, but this might not always be relevant to you, as the costs might not be displayed in ways that are relevant to your pocketbook.

WHO IS THE BEST SURGEON IN YOUR AREA? AN EXAMPLE

Let's break it down with an example. Say you are considering whether to get a knee replacement and you are wondering if there is any free information comparing orthopedists (bone surgeons) in your area.

I look up "orthopedics" on PhysicianCompare.com and it tells me, "There are 199 Healthcare Professionals related to 'orthopedics' within 5 miles of BALTIMORE, MD 21218." I look further down the list, and there are eighty-three physicians in the orthopedics category; unfortunately, there is little information available on how good any of them is.

Perhaps I should compare hospitals. Then I will pick the hospital that does the best job with knee replacements. So I go to 21218, my Baltimore ZIP code, and pick three hospitals to compare. The table won't be reproduced here, but you can go to the website and try putting in your own ZIP code.[3]

I noticed several things about the table that was presented to me. First, for one row, the rate of complications for hip/knee replacements, there is "no difference from the national rate" for the three hospitals I chose. Statistically speaking, this probably means that the difference between the hospitals is not larger than would be expected by chance and that one should not read too much into small differences. Of course, this raises a question regarding the national rate itself of 3.3 percent—that is, complications in three cases of one hundred—and whether this is a rate that you could tolerate as possible.

I also see that there is no data available on serious complications for the three hospitals I chose. Using publicly available information to decide which surgeon or hospital is better for me depends on that information being available in the first place. Similarly, there is no available information about deaths among patients with serious treatable complications after surgery. The headings on these two rows alone might raise fears and suspicions.

Your next step—until more data is available through federally mandated reporting—might be to seek out online recommendations from people. Which surgeons do they recommend? And why?

FINDING A SURGEON—OR SURGICAL OPTION— THAT'S RIGHT FOR YOU

Looking at the ratings available on Healthgrades.com, we see that they predominantly emphasize patient experience: ease of making appointments, courtesy and helpfulness of staff, waiting time, and the like. This matters to a lot of people, as can be seen by the mere number of ratings. But what if, in fact, you want to know about the rates of complications? Or the number of people who went to see a doctor and had an unsatisfactory result? What if you want to talk to the people who went to a surgeon and think they made the wrong choice way back when?

The ratings online tend to exclude people with negative experiences. The federal ratings systems tend to exclude those who find it hard to participate in surveys (the poor response rates of such surveys are a known phenomenon). The people who wish they hadn't chosen surgery in the first place likely are not going to share their comments about their experiences on the surgeon's ratings page.

This appears to be yet another area in which the research lags behind our real-world needs. What is the best way to find information about the full range of options for a condition for which surgery is commonly performed? There are plenty of diseases for which we all know that we should go to the emergency room, and there we might get surgery. For example, if we have terrible, acute abdominal pain, there is a chance it might be due to something wrong with one of the abdominal organs (the intestines, stomach, gall bladder, liver, kidney, spleen), and thus, in some cases, surgery might be a corrective.

There are many more cases in which surgery is one of multiple available options, and as we have seen, there is often no good evidence on whether, for us, the surgical option is the best one. To speak about a case in my clinic, Ms. X is a fifty-year-old woman with a PhD in the humanities and a diagnosis of sickle cell disease. Sickle cell can affect the body in different ways, and one of the ways is to affect the bones through a lack of blood supply: avascular necrosis. Avascular necrosis can cause significant pain, most commonly in the hips, and patients with sickle cell disease are those in whom this condition is not infrequently seen.

Unfortunately, Ms. X also has osteoarthritis (degenerative bone disease) in her hips. The combination of the arthritis and the avascular necrosis is quite disruptive to her. She lives an active life in her professional field, and because of her chronic pain, she has been on a number of medications over the years. Despite their potential habit-forming nature and the significant associated harms, she has taken chronic narcotics (opiates), which have been the only thing to control her pain. Nonetheless, by dint of determination, she has managed to decrease the dose of these medications little by little.

So she finds herself, as do the people in the other stories of this book, between a rock and a hard place. She is decreasing the dose of the narcotic medications she is taking because she is acutely aware of the associated harms. However, she still has her pain.

She has gone to the orthopedic (bone) surgeons to advise her on whether she should have surgery. Some do want to operate because they are confident that they can make a difference to her symptoms, and others do not, worrying that her avascular necrosis and her back pain may make it likely that her pain will not be significantly affected by a hip replacement.

Or take another patient of mine, Mr. L, a seventy-six-year-old man born in Panama. (He left Panama at the age of eighteen, when an American daughter of a military couple wooed him and convinced him to move to the United States with her.) He has chronic pain in his leg due to nerve damage (neuropathy) associated with diabetes. He also has a transplanted kidney. Every time he comes and sees me, he complains, legitimately, that his leg hurts. At some point, it was suggested to him that he see an orthopedist (bone doctor), which, to be honest, was not exactly my idea (though I did not oppose it). The orthopedic surgeon, to my great surprise, averred that he could substantially improve Mr. L's knee pain through a knee replacement.

Mr. L, his family, and I were faced with the task of how to approach the knee surgery. He was very hopeful that his pain could be significantly reduced, but I was not very sanguine, given the number of health issues he already had going on. His family was not sure and realized that I was skeptical; nonetheless, Mr. L was happy to go ahead. He had made his choice.

When we make a choice for surgery, what are we hoping for? Does Mr. L want to be pain free? That might be possible, but does he realize (even after I told him) that 10 percent of people still have long-term pain after knee surgery?[4] Does he want to be sure that he can participate in a wider range of physical activity? Or does he just want to be able to rely on the assurances of the surgeons and try the very hardest he can to achieve some sort of improved outcome? Is Mr. L, after all, just aiming for hope?

I am not acquainted with the deep roots of Mr. L's wish for surgery. (He is not the best communicator of his wishes, or perhaps I am not eliciting them very well, and the family members who come with him to appointments basically shrug and try to accommodate him.) But the possible grounds of Mr. L's wish for surgery make perfect sense when you consider how many people approach this decision, which is to talk to friends or family. Most people do not engage in the weighing of risks and benefits regarding the doctor they will see for their surgery or regarding whether they have a surgery. We might do ourselves a disservice if we demand an accounting of the criteria we use.

If Mr. L is not making a decision the way I would like him to make one—not consulting a website with figures and comparisons of rates—then how should he make the decision? In fact, I did ask him once how he was going about his decision making. Of course, I couldn't use that term, since that is not the way most of us talk. Indeed, I would bet that many of us do not think of our decisions as decisions; we have made the decision or come to a conclusion even before we come to see our doctor. But in this case, I asked Mr. L why he wanted to have the surgery. He said simply, "Because of the pain."

We could have tried to rewind the clock, Mr. L and I. I could have presented him with an annotated list of options and tried to discuss with him, in detail, the complications that might make surgery something to avoid (his age and the number of his already-existing medical conditions). I could have tried to engage his family with all of the pluses and minuses. To be honest, we did that, though one can always do a better job and it is not as if Mr. L was the type to come in with a list of detailed questions. However, in his heart of hearts, I think he had already made his decision before coming in and changing it was unlikely.

You are not Mr. L, just by the fact that you are reading this book. You are more engaged and aware. But the basic question still applies: When it comes to surgery, how can you be sure that you are making the correct decision?

I might have landed you in a dilemma. The scientific evidence is based on population and thus cannot afford a clear answer to you, as an individual, for whether you should be having surgery. And further down the chain of decisions, if you have settled on surgery as the option that is right for you, it is unclear whether there is sufficient data for you to be sure that you have picked the right surgeon.

One solution to this problem is to get more and more data, and certainly that is one route. For example, the precision medicine initiative recently promoted by President Obama foresees a large-scale cohort of about a million Americans who participate in research meant, on the basis of populations, to apply down to the level of individuals based on each person's genome. While your genetic makeup might not be relevant to the choice of surgery, the idea is that more data will help us get closer to the unique needs of the individual and the particular characteristics that might impact the choice of a given treatment—for example, surgery. Alternatively, as we discussed in the chapter on diabetes, a judicious use of Bayesian statistics might help us figure out which groups of patients are most likely to benefit from a given surgery.

But it is much more likely that what we might call "life factors" have a lot more to do with whether to have surgery and how to decide whether a particular surgeon is right for you. *Life factors* mean whether surgery *works* for you—that is, aligns with the constraints, desires, beliefs, and preferences you bring to other life choices. If I cannot ever tell you that surgery is the only possible choice for you, then you are the one who should make that decision, unencumbered by a sense that only the doctor is the one who can make that decision for you.

I think that the decision about which surgeon, which center, and what sort of surgery, while also affected by life factors, can respond to the body of evidence that has to do with surgical quality and safety. Pioneered by researchers such as Peter Pronovost, from my institution of Johns Hopkins, health-system researchers have focused on the qualities that make surgeries succeed.

One factor, which many people agree on, is volume. The more often a surgeon performs a procedure, the better she can become and the less likely it is that the patient will die soon after surgery.[5] While the parameters of this relationship are complicated and not without dispute (Does this apply to all procedures? Can a surgeon be an expert in a number of different procedures or only at one or two?), it seems uncontroversial that if you want an excellent open heart surgery, you go to the surgeon who has done them the most often. Whether you have access to the surgeon who has done the absolute most is another question, but if you have to choose between the more experienced and the less experienced surgeon, choose the more experienced one—that much seems clear.

But clearly that's not enough, because we all know situations in which the most experienced surgeon is just not the right one for us. In fact, as Mr. L's primary care doctor, I immediately had someone in mind, but that other surgeon had a booked schedule and could not fit him in. Thus, I had to refer him to another surgeon. And even if that surgeon has ample experience in the particular operation, there are other factors to consider.

NOT JUST THE MOST EXPERIENCED SURGEON

A distinction is commonly made between the surgeon with fantastic technical skills and a surgeon with a so-called bedside manner. Actually, the two go hand in hand.

My patient Ms. M is a seventy-one-year-old woman with chronic left leg pain who has the last stages of kidney disease. She dresses immaculately, usually in shades of off-white. Her husband died a few years ago, and while I think that sometimes she feels herself freer from the burden of caring for his many medical problems, she is lonely. Her several children tell her that she should move in with one of them, but she is certain that she wants to keep living alone. For a few years, she has been on the kidney transplant service, with the expectation that the transplant surgeon and his team would in time find her a new kidney. She would love to get a transplanted kidney because she knows that will grant her years of extra life compared to remaining on dialysis, which she is sick of and which makes her tired.

She does not make it to her appointments with perfect regularity because of her depression. However, she seems to take care of herself with surprising reliability given the number of her medical conditions and the chronicity of her left leg pain.

I have no doubt that the transplant surgeons she has seen are among the best anywhere, because the doctors at my institute are, in general, of high technical quality. However, in order to be evaluated for transplant at all, Ms. M has to be evaluated by the transplant team and conform to their conditions. Ms. M had been reachable only with difficulty on a number of occasions because she had been at dialysis whenever the surgery team tried to reach her.

Then I got a letter from the surgeons, and Ms. M got one at the same time. She was being put on their inactive list. This means that she would no longer be a candidate for transplant. I e-mailed the team to find out why this happened; the transplant coordinator, a nurse, responded promptly, but she did not know the details of the decision, which were determined at a meeting for the transplant surgeons, who themselves, at the time of the call, were not reachable (or, at least, did not respond to my e-mails).

Ms. M still wanted a transplant, and I referred her to another institution nearby. The question is not about the technical facility of either institution but about whether systems are in place to ensure a good outcome. If the systems assume that patients will shoulder the entire burden of follow up after a major operation—for example, transplant—then perhaps the systems are misguided and the surgeons who operate according to such a system are not to be preferred to surgeons who carry out their practice in another way. This doesn't make the surgeons bad people. It just means that their mode of practice is not to be relied on by us, and we shouldn't recommend them to others.

NEXT FRONTIER OF SURGERY: SYSTEMS OF CARE

Such systems of care, I think, are the next frontier in making sure that we are seeing the absolute best doctor for us (to the extent that is possible). On the one hand, we want a surgeon who is technically excellent, and that might be the surgeon who most often performs the procedure that we need. We would like a surgeon who is a good communicator, who is able to walk us through the risks and benefits attendant on a given procedure. However, we also want a surgeon whose practice organizes care in such a way as to make it accessible and relevant to us.

This means that if we decide to discuss the possibility of surgery, we should not feel railroaded into a decision. Of course, most surgeons would not do this. But we should not be abandoned into a decision, either; we should be provided with the names of patients who might be able to talk to us about their experiences. After the operation, we should be provided with specific advice about how to get our lives together and stories from other patients about what we can expect, not merely a referral to a physical therapist (though this can be very important as well).

In short, the perfect surgeon is not an individual but a collection of expertise, experience, and practice setting, together with the needs of the decision maker—that is, you. There is no perfection except what you need and what might work best for your situation.

9

HOW GOOD CAN GUIDELINES BE?

One of the greatest cognitive dissonances is found every single day in the doctor's or nurse's office. On the one hand, we go seeking care, whether it's an answer to our questions, reassurance that our lump or bump is not serious, guidance regarding a chronic condition, or relief of intractable symptoms. There are myriad reasons for our doctors' visits (or nurse visits), and many of them do not have anything to do with a particular medical symptom.[1]

In the office, we find the doctor or nurse. A human being, with their own biases and errors, their own style of practice. One doctor might be quite unlike another.[2]

Yet part of making doctors and health care better is trying to apply what we know best to daily practice—trying to let everyone know what works and avoiding what doesn't. To that end, groups of providers assemble regularly to create lists, directions, for how doctors (and, less often, nurses) should approach various circumstances of care. What is the best way to treat our blood pressure, diabetes, or heart disease? How should one care for a patient at the end of life? Is there a single best way to treat Lyme disease? Such are the questions that health care providers must deal with every day, and such directions, called guidelines, are an increasingly important part of health care.

Understanding how guidelines are made is like walking into a sausage factory—there's a little bit of everything; the process might not be appetizing; and there's no telling what might be left on the factory floor. But we have to put on our masks and helmets and venture into that space so that we can come out again, secure in the knowledge that these lists are imperfect, full of holes, and not necessarily relevant to what medical problems are like in daily life.

First of all, how is a guideline born? What makes a group of doctors (because they are mostly doctors) decide that authoring instructions for their colleagues is going to help matters?

Medical guidelines can be traced to the idea that care should be based on the best science and not individualized care growing out of the lore passed down from physician to physician or transmitted from colleague to colleague. By this account, guidelines are meant to assemble the best scientific evidence to help physicians in their decision making. Or, failing that, to present the evidence that is available to help physicians take account of its imperfections.

There are problems with this understanding of how guidelines are supposed to work. First, there is no perfect evidence that matters the same way to everyone, everywhere. On the contrary, it matters very much who is calling the information "evidence" and who is sitting in judgment upon it. One person's evidence might be another's trial with overly strict exclusion criteria, conducted among people who bear no resemblance to those suffering with the disease in question in the real world since women, children, the elderly, and those with common diseases are frequently excluded from such trials. [3]

Second, even if we accept that the process of guideline making can somehow connect the best scientific evidence to the care of patients, patients themselves are most often not involved in the process, though efforts are being made to improve this situation. [4] Imagine if a recipe were written without regard for how people might actually prepare it at home; we all know recipes that take, according to the expert chef, only twenty minutes of preparation time but in real life take closer to an hour. In a Platonic world of perfectly prepared recipes, they would be fit for the gods, but they would never make it onto the table of a real person.

Guidelines, like recipes, must be palatable to the end consumer.

Let's walk through some guidelines in order to understand how they are relevant, or not, to the actual day-to-day life of people with chronic conditions. Before we start, I should mention that these are the best of the lot. Guidelines, in general, have a multitude of problems, which we will address later, but first we should describe how they look in the best of circumstances and how applicable they might be to actual experience.

Most recently, doctors have taken notice of new guidelines for the treatment of cholesterol with medications known as statins. Such medications are widely used and are big business. You might have heard your doctor say that "everyone should be on a statin [cholesterol medicine] to prevent heart disease." Is this true? And where does this advice come from?

First, of course, the "everyone" is a red herring. I can't think of any medication that "everyone" should be on. (What would it be for, for starters? Not everyone is equally at risk for the same diseases, and the mix of risks and benefits is bound to be different for each patient. And what if each person were able to make an informed decision about whether the medication was right for them?) So that immediately makes the question more complicated: What would make it necessary for *me* to take a medication? What would flip the switch in my head?

For many, of course, that decision would lie in the authority of the physician, as imperfect as we know that to be. While many researchers and doctors agree that in order for care to be truly appropriate for and centered on the needs of the individual, it should consist of shared decision making (i.e., communication and decisions done together) much of the time this does not happen.[5] Often we can place the blame for this at the feet of the doctor or the system she works in—and we'll get to that below. Much of the time, however, it's also the patient who plays a role in making the visit unidirectional and ceding the decision to someone besides herself—usually because she is not comfortable making decisions; does not have the skills, education, or power needed to navigate the health care system; or is not aware that there are options to discuss and that she could, suitably empowered and engaged, take control.

HOW GUIDELINES ARE BORN

Whether or not you desire to make your decision in a partnership with a physician or want to adopt a traditional role where you learn the recommendations of an expert, it is important to know how guidelines are fashioned. The first step is to understand who is on guideline committees. There is no vetting process, or, rather, the way people ascend to be entrusted with the making of guidelines is the same way anyone rises to a position of power: through a combination of talent, luck, and time served.

This is not problematic in itself. There is no particular combination of talents, tendencies, and imperfections that fits one job best. There are successful doctors who have a poor bedside manner and great artists who are more organized than the average accountant. What is generally not checked in guideline development, however, is the conflicts of interest that may be obtained.

Conflicts of interest refer to any involvement that might, to an outside observer, appear to influence the judgments made in a set of guidelines. Most relevant, of course, are relationships to pharmaceutical or medical device companies. The physicians who serve on guideline committees tend to be the ones who are the most knowledgeable about their field. For most subfields of medicine, the type of knowledge that tends to be privileged is newness: new medications, new studies, new devices. And such newness can only be produced and promoted by companies with the money to do so.

Thus, the people who know most about whatever field is producing the guidelines (whether it be endocrinologists who treat diabetes and want to know which medication is the best in which circumstance; electrophysiologists who understand the conduction of electricity through the heart and which medications or procedures might restore the heart's rhythm in ways potentially beneficial to health; psychiatrists who treat depression and other mood disorders; physical therapists who try to get the body into working order after some sort of disorder; or another specialty altogether) tend to be the ones most invested in their particular specialty, their own institutionally and establishment-limited take on that disease.

It would be defensible, at this juncture, to decide that you do not need any of these specialists, given the imperfection of medical science, which we have pointed out here. It would be okay to be the sort of person who would like to make decisions based entirely on your needs and concerns, quite apart from what scientific or medical experts have decided is right for patients. Because you (or your loved one) is the patient. To express this in a circular way, the numbers only matter to you if . . . they matter to you. What does the blood pressure number matter if it doesn't make you feel better or—with a reasonable certainty—make it likely that you do not have a heart attack or stroke? What does the diabetes number (the hemoglobin A1C) number matter if, below a certain point, it does not guarantee any lower rate of heart attack, stroke, amputation, or kidney failure?

What is the point of taking a depression medication day in and day out if, on average, it makes you feel worse rather than better?

If you have knowledge of the treatments available to you, and they don't seem to work or align with your needs, then, by all means, do something else. However, many of us lack that knowledge. And that is one use for guidelines, issued by groups of doctors who are charged with deciding what information matters most for health decisions.

In any case, guidelines are complex and conflicted both intellectually and financially. Are they the best we have, or can we do better? Let's take a tour through the guts of one of them.

The statin guidelines are not named anything so simple; rather, they are the combined effort of the American College of Cardiology and the American Heart Association (sixteen authors, all told) under the formidable title "Guideline on the Treatment of Blood Cholesterol to Reduce Atherosclerotic Cardiovascular Risk in Adults."[6] (Here is a link to the article: http://content.onlinejacc.org/article.aspx?articleid=1879710.)

The guideline starts with its methodology, distinguishing it immediately as an enterprise of evidence-based medicine. We have talked about the weaknesses of this approach elsewhere. Peter Elias, a family doctor in California,[7] has said that he hates the term *evidence-based medicine* and prefers *evidence-informed medicine*. This is an abbreviated description of the distance we must travel between the evidence that undergirds such a guideline and the decisions we might, or might not, make with its help. It is not a simple matter of basing the medicine on evidence, in other words, but rather informing care with the evidence that we know to be imperfect.

The doctors charged with writing the guideline assembled a large number of studies, comparing patients who were on a medication for cholesterol to those who were not on a medication to see whether this medication influenced people's rates of heart attack, stroke, or other outcomes that people would like to avoid.

How do the researchers figure out which studies can be included in such a summary? What do they leave in or take out? And how do they pool the results of these studies in order to come up with a result that can inform guidelines? Can they ensure along the way that their methods are responsive to the needs of people who might be at risk for heart disease and are considering a cholesterol medication?

The so-called gold standard of scientific studies designed to assess medical treatments is the randomized controlled trial. Such a trial uses random numbers to assign patients to treatment or a control group, which, according to statistical theory, should make it more legitimate to compare the two groups of patients by equalizing the variables that have not been accounted for in designing the experiment. For example, if two groups are randomized and one group happens to have had a cholesterol medication sometime in the past, it is likely (if the second group is similar according to other characteristics) that the other group has as well.

In order to establish a statistically significant effect due to medication—that is, large enough so that it is not expected to be due to random chance—a certain number of patients is needed in a study. Such sample size is difficult to obtain without considerable government funding (it takes money to design a study, recruit patients, and analyze the data). More and more, given the limitations of such funding, studies are being supported by the same pharmaceutical companies that manufacture and market the very medications that are to be studied. To take the example of the ACC-AHA guidelines regarding cholesterol medications, the introduction states that "none of the ACC/AHA expert reviewers had relevant RW [relationships with industry]," with a link to appendix 2. A glance at appendix 2 shows that, in fact, six of the coauthors maintain relationships with industry in the form of consulting with a number of pharmaceutical and device companies. "Surely," the response might be, "it is unreasonable to expect cardiologists to maintain no relationships at all with these companies, especially when they are the ones that make the trials possible." In the current system this is precisely correct, but then one should also recognize what the potential downsides are to that system and what alternatives might exist. Moreover, one should consider whether "consulting" relationships are indeed of the kind that should be explicitly addressed whenever considering how reliable such a set of guidelines might be.

Be that as it may, these randomized controlled trials, as they are called, are placed at the top of the hierarchy when researchers summarize the results of different sorts of studies for their guidelines. Since these trials are difficult to fund, conceive, and carry out, and since the understandable tendency is to design trials that will find a statistically significant effect, the profile of a typical subject in these studies often does not jive with what we in the real world are like. That is to say, most often studies are done in a homogeneous population, often without chronic disease. However, since every person is different and the influence of other health conditions on our chance of being benefited by a cholesterol medication is often the question at issue, these studies often might not apply to us.

For this reason, perhaps other types of studies should be considered as top-quality evidence that a doctor might look at when making a recommendation, not just randomized controlled trials. These studies would include studies of patient experiences, cohort studies in which a group of patients is followed over time, case reports to understand the potential effects on a single patient, and so forth. The reason that a randomized controlled trial has been crowned the queen of study methodologies is that it, supposedly, can provide the most unbiased estimate of a population effect.[8] But when any one of us has to make a decision about whether taking a cholesterol medicine is right for us, we are not necessarily thinking about how effective the medication is in a population (though that is part of the information that many of us would like to have) but about how it is going to impact our life individually.

The main innovation of these guidelines had to do with their approach to the numerical value of the cholesterol test and how it matters (or, actually, doesn't matter as much as previous guidelines suggested). The previous iteration of this report suggested that the numerical value of cholesterol was important, and cholesterol medication should be titrated in order to fix cholesterol numbers. This is why so many of us still think that when we go to the doctor, we should get our cholesterol level checked regularly.

Here come the new guidelines and we find that there is no evidence to support the titration of cholesterol treatments based on cholesterol numbers. This makes sense, if only because other literature has shown us, since those previous guidelines, that cholesterol values can fluctuate significantly from day to day, even comparing day and night.[9] Furthermore, the supposed benefit of cholesterol medicines is to reduce the risk of heart attack and our death rates due to heart disease. So why not see if cholesterol medicine should instead be tailored to our level of such risk?

This is exactly the innovation of this new set of cholesterol-medication guidelines: to peg the recommendation for statin (cholesterol medication) not to the level of the cholesterol itself but to the estimated risk of heart disease.[10]

The trick, of course, is defining *risk* and "how much" the risk is actually reduced. Both of these are subject to dispute, which is not evident in the guidelines as promulgated—though, in fact, your doctor might dispute them herself (even if she might not make this obvious to you).

To be specific, one of the new elements of the guidelines concerning cholesterol medications is a risk calculator to estimate your risk of developing heart disease within the next ten years. The most famous of these was born of one of the first large-scale studies of heart disease, the Framingham study, based on a number of patients in Framingham, Massachusetts, who were followed over a number of years to see whether they developed heart disease. It is unclear how often physicians have actually used this previous calculator to estimate the risk of heart disease, though it is included in the decision aids online that are designed to empower us to make informed decisions about whether we would like to take a cholesterol medication.

The innovation in the new guidelines regarding the cholesterol medication is that a new value of risk was suggested to be "too" high—that is, high enough that someone with that level of risk would be "automatically" prescribed a cholesterol medication.

There are many things wrong with this approach. First, let us confine ourselves to the calculator itself. Many have pointed out that it consistently overestimates the cardiac risk for millions of Americans. Further, the risk of heart disease in the next ten years (as opposed to the next year or over an entire lifetime) is not an intuitive measure. [11]

The main problem, however, is in the algorithmic nature of these guidelines. How should we interpret them? Do we really follow doctors' guidelines according to their say-so, like a set of directions or a recipe?

It depends on how you see the role of the doctor in your life. While historically two possibilities have been most commonly propounded (either all-knowing sage or advisor to provide you with the tools to decide for yourself), in reality there is a spectrum of how we see the role of physicians and health care professionals in our lives. They can be sources of advice—impartial bearers of information, no matter how imperfect that information might be. They might be resources for further study of the question on our part. They can be goalposts to help us achieve our objectives. They might be our guides through a bewildering world of options, enabling us to make decisions for ourselves while respecting our values and preferences. [12]

This is where the algorithmic nature of a guideline like this one might be significantly frustrating to some of us. If we want a decision made by the doctor, fine, but shouldn't there be more consensus among doctors as to what is necessary? If we want the physician to be an old-school sage, dispensing advice, then shouldn't that advice be worth something? On the other hand, even if we want to make our own decisions, what is the point of the algorithm? Shouldn't we be able to do what we think is right and not be dropped into an algorithm like some sort of pinball?

The problem is, that the guidelines we are given are the only ones that exist. In other words, the process of guideline creation—the assembly of a specialized team of doctors, filtering the academic evidence to come to a conclusion that is supposed to apply algorithmically to a group of us, irrespective of our personal preferences—is unlikely to change. The mechanisms of academia, though they are beginning to include the voices of ordinary people more and more often, are steeped in a tradition of intellectual effort that views rigor with the highest esteem—even if that rigor, as we have stated before, is undermined by the very imperfections and biases of the evidence that is held up to be the highest standard.

There are various models for how to combine various sources of evidence, how to make medical and scientific endeavor applicable to our own daily lives. It is a real pity, a gap in the way doctors view the world, that guidelines such as those for cholesterol medicine do not include the views of ordinary people, patients. Indeed, there are many initiatives present in the world of patient engagement to include those views. Nevertheless, large-scale systemic change, upending the current hierarchical relationships between doctors, researchers, and patients, is still unlikely. We must figure out how to take these algorithms, these guidelines, and make them work for us.

One way to approach the statin guidelines as a special case of the problem of guidelines in general is more or less how they are conceived by the physicians who assemble them. That is, approach the question about whether to use the cholesterol medication depending on the cardiac risk that the risk calculator estimates for you. You enter your blood pressure, last cholesterol values, presence or absence of diabetes, smoking, and previous heart attack, and out comes an estimate of your heart-attack risk over the next ten years. [13]

A couple of provisos should be attached to these directions. First, the decision aids fashioned on the basis of these guidelines direct that a patient should not use them without the advice of a doctor. Whether to respect this admonition depends on how you see your relationship with your doctor or whether you have a primary care doctor or nurse at all. For those without a health care giver, these online decision aids, based on guidelines, provide a potential resource that is not dependent on fragmented, often still-unaffordable primary care.

Second, the risk calculator is quite vehemently disputed in scientific circles. This calculator, as mentioned above, differs from the previously widely used version in the population that was used as the base for defining the mathematical model that, in turn, estimates the risk of heart disease. It also differs, as said above, in the cutoff used to define those at increased risk, suggesting that all people with a ten-year risk of heart disease of 7.5 percent be prescribed statins, the cholesterol-lowering agents.

The objections raised against this guideline up to now have mostly been focused on the fact that lowering the cutoff for "high" risk will, presumably, lead millions more of us to take anticholesterol medications.[14] (Leaving aside that such recommendations do not necessarily lead to us taking the medications we are prescribed, which is another topic entirely. For example, many people with hypertension do not have it sufficiently controlled with medication—about 40 percent of men and 60 percent of women.[15]) But another major repercussion of the new guidelines, which has not been addressed as much in the scientific literature, is that it exposes millions more people to algorithmic care.

There is nothing wrong with algorithmic care if that is what you prefer. But the guideline, as written, does not include a commonsensical suggestion: that patients be asked about their preferences in how such guidelines should be applied to their care. (A "risk discussion" is encouraged, but that is not the same thing.[16]) If you are that sort of person who would like to take a treatment according to the way it might modify your risk of heart disease, then all is well and good, though you might like to be informed about the uncertainties inherent in any scientific estimate of such risk. If, however, you might like to make your own decision about whether to take the medication, even after being informed about the risk, you should be able to do that, too. Or, finally, if you would like to take a completely different approach to the treatment of your cholesterol, that possibility does not seem to be recognized by the guidelines as currently laid out.

The guidelines, in short, are to help doctor and patient answer the question: Should the patient be taking a cholesterol medication? This supposes that asking questions about potential decisions is the right way to approach a health care problem. But there are many ways, outside of decisions, to approach a risk for heart disease. One is medication; one is nonmedication routes to treatment; and another is a decision that a risk for heart diseases of whatever magnitude is not sufficient to motivate taking a medication on the basis of incomplete scientific evidence that might not apply to the individual.

In other words, when a doctor says, "You need to be on a cholesterol medication," consider the risks and benefits of that medication and also consider, quite apart from any algorithm, whether that particular balance works for you and your life. That is the only right answer.

10

IS HALF OF ALL RESEARCH WRONG?

Part of the reason we go to doctors is to benefit from their expertise. We want the advice of someone who knows better than we do. Even given the recent moves of health care in the direction of shared discussions between us and our doctors, we still go to someone who we think possesses information, experience, and specialized training that we do not. Somewhere in the back of our minds we think that medicine is based on scientific research. Medical scientists go out and find the truth, and then—allowing for some inexactitudes and imperfections—it can be applied to our physical or mental health. The doctor's job is to take that science and bring it to the benefit of our health.

What if the science itself is less true than we thought? Or, rather, what if the process of doing science introduces uncertainties that make it inapplicable to our individual cases?

Examining the process of medical science—how the findings are arrived at, how they are checked and published, and how they are brought to bear on individuals—can help us answer this question.

We start with the definition of *science*, which seems like an impossibly ambitious goal. To avoid the entire philosophical tangle, I will say here that science is the collection and analysis of information supported by infrastructures. Surely there is much effort devoted to learning the proper methodology, which information to collect and how, and, even before that stage, how to precisely define the scientific questions to ask of the data. But in the context of applying science to the care of the individual patient, the context of science—the structures that support it and the incentives that people follow—matters just as much as the elements that people consider intellectual.

Let us take hypertension as an example. Previously, I have referred to a systematic review that was recently done in the *Annals of Internal Medicine* showing a benefit to the treatment of mild hypertension. Such a systematic review aims to combine the results of multiple randomized controlled trials.

Now we need to explain each term I just used in order to come to an understanding of how scientific methods are themselves determined by the societal incentives that give rise to science.

Trials cost money to conduct, though the literature on the costs of studies of antihypertension medication seems thin. In order for these trials to be successfully conducted, they are usually limited to those subjects whose preexisting diseases will not muck up the works. That is, people with a number of other diseases might not even be included in the studies that attempt to assess the effectiveness of a given medication, because there is concern that their other diseases either will reduce the effectiveness of the tested medications or will increase the potential harms.

Second, the "outcomes"—that is, the results that the antihypertension medicines are supposed to prevent—might differ from trial to trial. How do researchers decide on what outcomes to look at for a given medical treatment? Do we prefer that a medication reduce death or disease? Improve quality of life? Is affordable to take and does not unfavorably interact with our other medications? Is not associated with intolerable side effects or potential harms?

Obviously, one answer is the most serious damage that a disease can do to us. Blood pressure can kill and can cause increased rates of heart attack, stroke, and kidney failure. Thus, it would stand to reason that a study about hypertension medications should look at these as potential outcomes. Unfortunately, it takes years of following patients in a study for enough of them to develop these outcomes to make analyzing the findings of the study possible statistically.

Therefore, these outcomes are occasionally combined in so-called composite outcomes, which make it more feasible to conduct the complicated, expensive trials without having to recruit more patients by an order of magnitude. Unfortunately, these outcomes make the findings less relevant to people who take these medications. Avoiding a heart attack makes sense, as does avoiding a stroke, but who thinks about avoiding "any combination of bad things"?

The problem of outcomes that are relevant to us is being addressed by the Patient-Centered Outcomes Research Institute (PCORI), a federally funded agency designed to center research around things that actually matter, not only to researchers but also to ordinary people.[1]

The problem extends well beyond just the definition of *outcomes*. How do we know that a result arrived at in a trial is true? How can we tell whether the result of such a scientific study is applicable to our own lives? Do the answers to these questions have anything to do with each other?

Many recent books introducing the public to the rudiments of statistical analysis have described how statistical analysis is supposed to work, how noise is sifted for data.[2] There is a basic and important distinction between those who see data as randomly distributed, with exceptions that experimental science is meant to ferret out, as opposed to data as representative of a number of potential hypotheses, with an experiment able to distinguish between them.

Recent controversy has erupted in the scientific community around the ways in which signal is selected from the noise. Are studies "rigged" in advance to aim at the tests of statistical significance that will get them published? Are comparison groups, populations studied, and outcomes chosen merely for the sake of publication? If so, then a bias is involved, and the truth-seeking nature of medical science is in question.

Our response to this should not be surprise that bias afflicts the scientific literature (it is a human enterprise and thus afflicted by such bias), nor should we be shocked—or determined that we will throw out the whole of the scientific enterprise. That would be going too far. Rather, we should use knowledge of the way science is done, and its very real imperfection, as a guide to help us fill in the research gaps—not in the distant future, but now and for us.

Back to the claim that is the title of this chapter. In order to understand how research is conducted and what that means for our help, we should consider a basic question: How do we know if research findings are true?

One method to see whether research findings are due to a "new finding"—that is, something we did not believe before—on the one hand, or merely a random collection of chance observations, on the other, which is called *frequentist statistics*. In brief, we estimate the probability that the data we see as the result of a study is due to chance or due to our previous belief (the "null hypothesis") being rejected.

However, for a variety of reasons, the "probability values," or p-values, reported in scientific journals do not represent the true likelihood that the set of data is appreciably different from chance. This is because researchers tend to report data that meets the statistical criteria for significance (that is, data that is sufficiently different from chance to point to some needed change in hypothesis) and are likely not to report as assiduously data that does not meet those criteria. Further, there is publication bias, in which only those publications that meet the criteria of statistical significance tend to get published, leaving those journal articles that do not establish a finding to languish unread in computer files or desk drawers. Finally, there are problems with study designs themselves: the outcomes, participants, and interventions (the treatment that is given to the participants in the study), such that these are tailored to arrive at publishable results.

In essence, the problems with studies, what has led various biostatisticians to debate to what extend the findings of journal articles are true, are the same problems with the application of the studies to our health care. The lessons from populations are not easily reducible or extendible to our particular case—not just because we are different from any population (we are unique), or because we don't agree with the science (we have our own thoughts and are autonomous), but also because the science itself is not aiming unerringly at truth but somewhere off to the side.

There are various approaches to this problem. The first is to better define just how often, and to what extent, the statistical analyses of scientific articles do not arrive at the truth. This was the purpose of John Ioannidis's paper on this topic, which became deservedly famous.[3] Deservedly so, because it was one of the first papers to lucidly ask the question: Given sources of bias in the research literature, how sure can we be that a result reported with statistical significance is actually true? And what does this mean for the medical literature in particular? Ioannidis used a model and a set of assumptions to estimate the extent of bias in the extant scientific literature.

What if these assumptions are wrong, however? Recently, two biostatisticians, Leah Jager and Jeffrey Leek, took another step, sampling thousands of scientific abstracts to see whether their results were most likely true. While this also involved assumptions about the likelihood that particular sets of data are found in a given range, it was based on empirical data from these thousands of abstracts—comparing, that is, the range of their "probability values" to the range that would be expected under particular ranges of the truth. Jager and Leek's work showed that, in fact, "half of all research is wrong" is possibly the upper range of the true estimate of falsity of the scientific literature.[4]

This means that more scientific papers are true than we might have thought.

Now we are again in a spot. Even if the most accurate estimate of the "false discovery rate" of published scientific articles is actually not as bad as 50 percent but still 17 percent or so (as was estimated by Jager and Leek), we still don't know what to make of each individual study—whether it applies to us, or whether the results it arrives at are true at all (or at least "true enough").

If that's the case, maybe there is a way to combine individual studies so that we can get a reliable, thirty-thousand-foot view of the scientific literature. Such pooling of results might enable us to figure out which results to rely on, which to ignore, and, in sum, to fashion a sort of average that could apply to as many people as possible.

There is, in fact, a heavily relied upon branch of epidemiology that does just this, and one I have been involved with for the past few years. It tries to review the body of peer-reviewed scientific literature with a priori algorithms for the identification of research questions: Which population is being studied? Which comparison is being made—that is, if we are trying to see which of x or y is better, which exact comparison are we making and why? What is the outcome we are interested in, and is it relevant? What is the time frame of the comparison we are looking at? And, finally, what is the setting in which this comparison is brought to bear?

This part of epidemiology is called *systematic reviews*, and I have been helping carry them out as part of a federally funded center at Johns Hopkins, supported under the auspices of the Agency for Healthcare Research and Quality. According to some views of the "evidence hierarchy" of evidence-based medicine,[5] a systematic review is one of the most reliable forms of scientific evidence, combining the results of multiple randomized controlled trials into a more globally applicable finding.

Indeed, when doctors get together to fashion recommendations, or guidelines, for their colleagues, they often rely on such systematic reviews of the peer-reviewed medical literature.[6] These are better than individual trials and certainly better than mere narrative driven by the biased experiences of experts—or so the theory goes.

From what we have seen about the difficulty of applying trials to our personal experiences, however, the claims made about systematic reviews as the most reliable form of evidence should give us pause. First, because each individual trial involves limitations in the population, comparison, and outcomes (one or more of these might not be applicable to our given case). It would be wonderful if combining these trials would fill the holes of generalization, enabling us to apply the findings to ourselves in particular.

Sometimes it does happen this way, and systematic reviews can serve important functions. However, more often than not, reviews of trials with holes in them lead to a big block of studies with holes. The holes can be extensive enough so that they connect to each other, so to speak, in a kind of Swiss cheese—their limitations overlap until it is not clear to whom they apply.

I will give an example appropriate to a patient of mine. Ms. L is a fifty-three-year-old woman who had bypass surgery in 1998 and thereafter has had two stents placed in her heart arteries. She was recently hospitalized for chest pain, and while she was not having an actual heart attack (in which heart muscle dies due to a lack of blood flow), we agreed it was most likely that her ongoing symptoms were due to a decrease of blood flow to her heart.

Such angina is certainty not an uncommon diagnosis, and much ink has been spilled in the scientific literature about how to treat it.

Ms. L came to me, in a follow-up visit after her hospitalization, with one simple question: What was it that had caused her chest pain, and what were we going to do about it in the future? We talked about angina and how to prevent it. Luckily, she was already on a number of good medications, but her further question was: How could we improve her medication regime? What should be added, subtracted, or changed?

She is already on a number of common medications to treat angina: a beta-blocker (which reduces the heart rate and the "squeeze" of the heart as it pumps, reducing the work of the heart, its blood requirement, and thus the pain) and a long-acting nitrate—that is, the same medicine as in the nitroglycerin pills put under the tongue but in a longer-duration form. Also, part of her regimen is Lisinopril, a member of the angiotensin-converting-enzyme (ACE) class of medications. She is trying to lose weight and engage in more physical activity; she does not have any chest pain now, but she would like to make sure that she is on the absolute best medications to treat her angina.

Naturally, she and I took a moment to talk about what the scientific literature shows about treatments for angina. The first thing we took note of was that the literature has not been much replenished in recent years with a comparison of already-existing treatments. There have been multiple recent studies on alternative therapies for angina—for example, gingko biloba and acupuncture. We did not discuss these alternative treatments, though perhaps we should have, if only to review the lack of evidence of their effectiveness in angina.

Another thing to notice is that the trials of angina treatment, besides being dated, generally compare one treatment to another rather than combinations of treatments. (There are statistical techniques to create such combinations indirectly even if they were not compared directly in a study; one is called *network meta-analysis*.[7] However, at the time of this writing, I am not aware of any such analysis for the medications that are meant to treat angina.) Moreover, the new medications are not compared to old medications but to placebo. And the outcomes, as mentioned above, are defined so as to be assessable from a statistical point of view and do not necessarily reflect how we would see our condition.

But the question every one of us should ask is not just "Are the results of these studies generalizable to me as an individual?" but also "Are they true?" Do they make sense in the world we live in? When we are talking about medicine, the truth of a research study is more than the statistical significance of the result and more than whether the data fits one hypothesis more than the other.

It has to do with the distinction between science and practice and what turns medicine into health care.

Medical science is a creature of the scientific establishment. I do not use the term *establishment* pejoratively. Science is a complicated enterprise and requires copious amounts of funding, expertise, and organization. The resources required to study the physiology of the heart, the structure of its muscles, the way the cells work and the ions flow through their membranes to get the large pump moving, and then the way in which the blood can be blocked in the heart vessels, causing pain—all of these things are basic human endeavors and rightly require massive support.

Determining whether research results are true as they relate to the heart, the way it pumps, how its cells move, and the potential blockages of blood on its way through the vessels is a completely normal scientific enterprise—albeit not a simple question. Philosophers of science tie themselves in knots trying to explain why it is, on the one hand, that the laws of science seem to jive with an observable reality, and why it is, on the other hand, that our understanding of that reality seems to change throughout the centuries—and not in a steady march of progress but in a sine curve, up and down; now in one direction, now in another.

In other words, is reality discovered by scientific laws (are the laws mapping out nature that is already there?), or is scientific research less like cartography than sculpture, shaping a figure that bears some relationship to the figure of reality? Or is reality too manifold and complicated and changeable with time to ever be depicted by science?

You can pick either alternative, but when it comes time to talk about something different from biomedical science (and different from the population science of public health—that is, individual health care), you are no longer in the realm of science. Here you are in the realm of practice, or phronesis, which is something else entirely.

Practice is meant not to arrive at a representative result, an aesthetically pleasing whole, a predictive model, a statistical representation of states of affairs, or an expansion of the bounds of knowledge. It is meant to arrive at a kind of action that represents or is structured by a moral outlook, a wisdom in determining ends and the means to attain them.

If the aim of medicine is such a practice—not a description of reality but ways to get to desired outcomes—then perhaps it is not so different from the aims of clinical trials and other common methodologies of biomedical science. Indeed, trials, as well as other kinds of peer-reviewed scientific literature, are trying to identify the best treatment, the best diagnostic technologies, and so on.

As we have seen, however, the design of such trials makes them more akin to scientific investigations, in which the aim is to determine the answer to a well-defined question or to arrive at a particular model of reality. Factors are isolated until a particular interaction or effect of a single medication or a single symptom is the object of the study at hand. The scientific enterprise is meant to establish causality. In Ms. L's case, the causal question would be, for example, whether the medication we were discussing at her visit, the calcium-channel blocker known as amlodipine, would reduce symptoms of angina in a given population.

In such a study, a population would be carefully selected, most likely through research volunteers at one of multiple medical centers. These volunteers would most commonly be taken from academic practices, though more and more often studies are being run under the auspices of private industry. Then, based on criteria devised prior to the study, patients who are too sick, have too many health problems, would not be able to understand sufficiently to participate, or could not speak English (in most studies done in the United States) would be excluded from the study. At this point, even after these criteria, Ms. L would theoretically still be included.

The study that is lacking is patients like Ms. L—in their fifties, with angina that has more or less been stable, without a heart attack or another problematic development, but has recently worsened—who already are on multiple medications for angina. What should Ms. L do? Should she drop the ACE inhibitor and start the calcium-channel blocker? Should she risk the side effects that go along with amlodipine? And how is she to know how her symptoms might respond?

There is no clear answer to these questions. Most likely, Ms. L will have to make some kind of decision. It might be enough to rely, as many doctors do, on some notion of experience with which alternatives work for certain patients and not for others. Maybe your doctor had a patient who did well switching from an ACE inhibitor to a calcium-channel blocker. Or maybe Ms. L is particularly worried about the common side effect of edema that is associated with the medication amlodipine. Or, even more practically, perhaps Ms. L's insurance, for whatever reason, covers one class of medications and not another.

If that is the case, if there is no study that precisely addresses Ms. L's question, then the question of "what is true" evaporates into the ether, and we are left with "what is good enough." And this question about good enough in the setting of particular practicalities and limited evidence is the basis of the practice of medicine.

What would it look like to search for "truth" in the setting of the practice of health care to benefit patients like Ms. L?

It would shift the definition and emphasis of the scientific enterprise, at least in the way in which it touched individual patients. It would try to answer the questions: What works best for patients in this situation? Are there situations for which there is evidence in the literature to which we can analogize Ms. L's question? What treatment goals matter for Ms. L, and what kind of approach works for them?

There are already research methodologies that have such an emphasis. They are classified as "qualitative," which is supposed to be opposed to "quantitative." Quantitative, obviously, is meant to focus on things that can be counted, and qualitative, by contrast, is supposed to focus on narratives or on the particular characteristics of things. This dichotomy is an oversimplification. Because what to count, as we have seen, requires a particular conception of what counts—and what is not countable is sometimes the very essence of understanding.

Ms. L's problem might best be understood through such qualitative methods. Which medicine is best added to other medicines or taken away? What are the possible experiences of patients who have gone through this situation?

The studies are not going to compare the particular combination that is relevant to Ms. L, but the experiences of other patients might inform her decision.

What should Ms. L actually do, though, while she is waiting for a realignment of our research priorities and until we gather the evidence necessary to compare the experience of different kinds of patients who make various choices regarding their regimens of angina treatments, including different kinds of medications? In the meantime, Ms. L found it more comforting to rely on the directive advice of her cardiologist, one of my Johns Hopkins colleagues. There will always be such situations in which the personal question outpaces the available scientific evidence. Until then, some stop gaps might be available.

We should search on the Internet and on social media for the numerous support groups that are available to help us make sense of our illness and to provide us with examples of people who have had to make similar decisions.

Customarily, doctors warn patients to stay away from such data, since it is not scientific and not validated in the peer-reviewed literature. However, as we have seen, since the peer-reviewed literature itself often does not apply to an individuals' uniqueness or particular question, we have to rely on some individual-level data. For reasons of generalizability (so we are not depending solely on one individual's story but a larger number of people), we would like to have recourse to databases of patients who are suffering problems like us. Failing that, however, our doctors are likely to recommend that we listen to their advice rather than those of other patients, because, as the theory goes, their experience is more reliable than laypeople's opinions.

However, if there's one thing that we know thanks to evidence-based medicine, it's that the personal experience of physicians is not notably reliable. Doctors only see their own particular, small slice of the population, which might not be representative of our situation at all—and they are not in our situation, that of the patient.

Thus, the best approach to the likely significant fraction of wrong or inapplicable research is not to make everything right again by refashioning the research and clinical systems we live in, at least not in the short term, but to use such inapplicability and wrongness as a pivot to focus on our own individual needs and concerns.

11

AVOIDING FALSE CERTAINTY AND APPROACHING FUTURE EXPERIENCES

"**W**hat's going to happen to me, Doctor?" said Ms. H.

She had just received some bad news from me, this African American woman in her fifties who had come to me a few weeks ago with tingling in her feet and new pain in her abdomen. She didn't know what was causing it and figured I would chalk the whole thing up to stress. In fact, I nearly did, but I checked some blood tests first.

The blood test showed that her blood sugar was 529 (normal is 125 or less). Her glycohemoglobin, a measure of the amount of sugar-bound blood cells, was 15 percent.

That is, she had a new diagnosis of diabetes. When she saw me at first, diabetes was not high enough on my list of suspicions to try and prepare her for such a diagnosis.

What were we going to do now? First, I asked about her experience with diabetes in her family. She had a sister living with diabetes who had not been able to get many of her medications or any consistent treatment (perhaps due to financial reasons; it was not clear why); she had a father who passed away recently, though she said not due to diabetes.

But then she wanted to know the answer to the most important question of all for her: What was going to happen to her? What life would she have and what could she expect?

At that moment, I wasn't sure what to answer.

There are things that patients might expect to hear from doctors. "Everything will be all right" is something I have caught myself about to say more than once. The phrase was formed in my mind and it was just about to be uttered until I realized that, in fact, I didn't know whether everything would be all right with her.

Unfortunately, and I should have predicted this, it was precisely this question that she asked me next. But not in those words.

"I don't think I have diabetes," she said, "because I am not ready to accept that diagnosis."

How could I predict what might happen to her if she herself wasn't sure that she had diabetes in the first place?

This question might seem ridiculous to those with a predominantly scientific conception of medicine. Claims about diagnosis and treatment are either true or not—they don't depend on the patient's opinion!

But medicine is a practice and depends on the interaction between patient and doctor. If Ms. H is told she has diabetes but does not accept the diagnosis, then it may be more difficult to figure out what treatments might work for her.

Additionally, the course of untreated diabetes is difficult to predict. (The most effort has been devoted to understanding how kidney disease due to diabetes might progress with time.[1]) There are those who can live years without any evidence of eye disease, problems in their leg arteries or veins, or heart disease.

The scientific literature about diabetes is one of the broadest on any medical topic. It includes a number of population studies tracking how the disease might develop in certain groups of patients with diabetes. However, the focus of this literature is, in my opinion and that of many others, misplaced. Instead of diabetes as it affects the individual, a molecular measure of glycohemoglobin, the hemoglobin A1C, is emphasized. And too-certain advice is given to people based on that literature. Even the National Institute of Diabetes and Digestive and Kidney Diseases, a reliable source of information, says on its website that "studies have shown that people with diabetes can reduce the risk of diabetes complications by keeping A1C levels below 7 percent."[2] However, there is controversy on that score; whether numerical targets should be the goal of diabetes treatment is more and more widely discussed.[3]

"The hemoglobin A1C should be lower than 7.5 in people in your age range," we hear from our doctor. Then we ask, reasonably, why that is. And perhaps the answer we get is something like "if you can control your sugar in that range, you can prevent certain health consequences."

This supposes a degree of certainty which is not actually the case.

In case after case, we are told that if we don't do such and such, something will happen. Or if we behave in this or another way, we will be able to prevent disease.

This advice is well intentioned; doctors want to help, and the idea that we can control our health care futures through our actions is sometimes plausible and even true. But there are plenty of actions whose consequences cannot be predicted.

Take smoking, which probably every doctor will universally tell you is something that you need to quit. Smoking confers a much-increased risk of lung disease, heart disease, and cancer. So if you stop it, you are free from these things, right?

If I have learned anything from using Twitter and other social media, it is that everyone has their own stories, and they do not always follow the cause-effect relationships that we are led to expect.

So there is Mr. C, a physicist, who developed colon cancer at the age of thirty-five despite the lack of family history and living a "blameless," healthy life. And there is my patient who is seventy-five and has been smoking for the past twenty years. Everyone has stories like this, and then the typical doctorly response is, well, that is true of populations, but you don't know if you are going to be the one affected.

Here I want to think about certainty, uncertainty, and health care. Is there any response to this conundrum of not knowing what will happen to us as individuals even if we have some degree of certainty about trends in populations?

In reading the scientific literature and meeting lots of patients and doctors who struggle with uncertainty, I have come up with some ideas. This chapter is more in the nature of a quasi-manifesto than a strictly rigorous scientific examination, because the notion of the overcertainty of biomedicine as currently presented is, unsurprisingly, not likely to be commonly treated in the peer-reviewed scientific literature. However, this overcertainty is an issue that will not go away as long as we are focused on medicine not as a practice but as a science reaching after truth.

Before we talk about some ideas to mitigate the effects of false certainty, why does it matter?

First, because it makes us less likely to question the advice of our doctors or other health care providers. Since, as outlined elsewhere in this book, health care providers might be as prone to make mistakes and suffer cognitive biases as the rest of us, asking fewer questions will get us into trouble.

Second, because if doctors think they are operating under certainty—if they are scientists and not practitioners—they will be more likely to make mistakes. This is found in other hierarchies as well, the disinclination to correct error when one thinks it has been eliminated from the system or does not consider it at all.[4]

Third, because practice requires a different model than certainty, as Annemarie Moll addressed in her book *The Logic of Care*.[5] Certainty requires an asymptotic striving toward the truth—ever onward, ever closer; if we are not there yet, then eventually, or at least theoretically, we will get there.

But uncertainty requires a different approach: we are going to do the best we can with the materials available to us at the moment.

Here are possible strategies to help you react to uncertainty in the context of your health based on patients I have known and perhaps relevant to your stories as well.

First, you can figure out what outcome matters to you. If there is no definitive certainty about the scientific evidence—for example, if you have hip osteoarthritis, you might know that recent trials have shed doubt on the universal effectiveness of physical therapy[6]—then you might have to engage in some trial and error in order to find a treatment that works for you. And "working" is going to be according to your definition, not the one decided on in scientific trials, even if your doctor might be less comfortable with your definition than with the "scientific" one. Similarly, when you discuss your health with your provider and try to figure out what treatment might work for you, you should come up with criteria (before you embark on a course of treatment) to help you decide when a given attempt will be enough. While we know from cognitive psychology that people, due to their inborn biases, tend to "discount" (underestimate) the benefit that certainty therapies might bring to them, such bias can be counteracted through carefully considering things in advance.[7]

Other options are to have other goals besides certainty, even other goals outside the individual objectives that matter to you. If you are interested in founding your care on a broad-based empirical approach to health, you might choose one of several topics that have received consistent attention and represent potential ways of organizing health care options in a way that might help both you and your community.

As I write these words, people are protesting in the streets of Baltimore because of ongoing police brutality on the part of the Baltimore Police Department. This is not an isolated issue with the use of police forces, however, but a demonstration of inequity in the way that the city systems are organized and paid for. Owing to a long history of institutional segregation, health care also is unfairly distributed in Baltimore and other cities. [8]

Does your own care as an individual have anything to do with this discrimination? And what does that have to do with avoiding a false chase after certainty?

In the current biomedical paradigm, "science" as an organizing principle for our health care helps give us confidence that we are treated according to the best available evidence. In the absence of such total certainty, perhaps we can choose from other governing philosophies that also might lead to improved care for us and others.

In response to the events that are occurring as I write, one possibility is to advocate—for oneself and for others—for equitable health care.

Let me explain the connections between freeing oneself from false certainty and advocating for equal health care for all. According to the present biomedical paradigm, as I explained earlier, health care is to be approached as a science. There is one truth, and research will find it; there is a best medication for hypertension or perhaps best treatments for subclasses of people. Similarly, there is a best glycemic target—the best level of the hemoglobin A1C value, to which diabetes control should aspire. The goal for arthritis should be to repair the joint, and this goal should apply to everyone.

But if such certainty is not to be our goal, because we realize the limits of science and the different needs of each individual, we find ourselves at a space where each person needs to be provided the best of health according to their own needs and preferences.

Thus, decreasing health disparities—making sure everyone gets whatever health services they need without regard to race, economic status, sexual orientation, or other characteristics—go hand in hand with making sure we do not automatically assume there is a certain medical truth out there.

But avoiding certainty means more than decreasing disparities; it means figuring out what is most important to you in your health. For that reason, understanding what your neighborhood and community need are essential in order to take account as counterweights to the biomedical paradigm. If, for example, there is no perfect treatment for high blood pressure, no one medication that works the best for every individual, then in order to maximize the dimensions of health that matter most to you in this instance (would you prefer to optimize diet and exercise rather than take a medication that might be associated with unpredictable side effects?), you might have to work with your community or neighborhood to make it happen. For instance, exercise is more difficult when safe, accessible walking routes are not available; diets are difficult to make healthy when fruits and vegetables are not easily obtainable.

Further, if the biomedical paradigm does not direct us to one solution for each health problem, then we need to find other dimensions to guide us. To continue with the example of the hypertension treatment, if we are not sure which medication is best for us—and the available literature does not suggest one optimum treatment—then we have to choose among other factors important to us in our lives. Do we want to take a medication or not, for example?

It is taken as gospel by some doctors of my acquaintance that hypertension should be treated by medication. However, there are many other options, as the hypertension chapter in this book discusses, such as physical activity, diet, and careful monitoring.

Becoming aware of the complete spectrum of treatment options for each health problem is the way to integrate one's own personal preferences and avoid the false assumption of uncertainty. In general, the assumption that "if there is a treatment, it should be used" is one to question.

It could be that the treatments are associated with harms that are unknowable or greater in significance for the given individual than their potential benefits. It could be that the person to whom treatment is suggested is just not the type to pursue treatment. Or it could be that the potential patient is burdened with distrust of the health care system so that he or she does not feel comfortable pursuing treatment within it.

Which sort of person would that be who wouldn't want treatment? That is what medicine is here for, to help people who need it!

I WOULD PREFER NOT TO

More and more often in my practice, I have started noticing patients who would prefer not to be treated. I have not seen this phenomenon addressed or exhaustively documented in the peer-reviewed literature, but I will try and make a start here, unscientific as it may be.

Mr. B is a religious Muslim man from Long Island who travels a considerable distance to see me in Baltimore, though I have told him there are plenty of doctors in New York City for him to see. Five years ago, he was diagnosed with kidney cancer and had a kidney removed. Recovering from that, he had a very large gastrointestinal bleed. After all this, he continued a career as a financial adviser, though, due to the general weakness of the economy and the barriers he had to overcome as a gentleman in his sixties with chronic health conditions, he was still relatively impoverished.

About a year and a half ago, he was diagnosed with a thoracic aortic aneurysm—that is, an outpouching in his abdominal aorta. At a certain diameter, the risk of such an aneurysm rupturing, or bursting, becomes more significant, and thus current practice is for surgery to be recommended when that size is reached.

He was first diagnosed with the aneurysm before he started seeing me as his doctor and had already begun regular monitoring of the aneurysm with CT scans—not an exceptional thing to be done.

At some point, his aneurysm started getting larger. It was not yet six centimeters in diameter, but the diameter was increasing by a tenth of a centimeter every six months or so. He was feeling well, or at least as he had felt for the past few years (weak, but still able to work, with the accompaniment of chronic pain). In that period, he came to me every few months, partially for the refill of his pain medications but also to discuss his aneurysm and whether, and with whom, it should be repaired.

On the one hand, he has always told me he wants it repaired, and I have no reason to doubt that this is what he *means to tell me* that he wants. That is, he thinks that he needs to tell me that he wants the surgery, and he is very conscientious about the pros and cons of the different surgeons he is considering—more detail oriented and conscientious than many patients in the same situation.

Time after time, or, rather, visit after visit, he wants to postpone the decision about surgery. He gives an excellent reason, which is important to his own circumstance: he is very worried (given his medical problems and the potential risk of any surgery) that he might die during the surgery and his wife (who, in addition to working full-time herself, has been assiduously helping take care of her husband's many medical issues) would be left without a means of support.

Since he cannot bear the thought of that happening, he tells me, he would like to wait to have the surgery done so that he can have a "nest egg" saved up before the surgery. Except his employment is not stable.

In the meantime, he has switched to another job and—given the expenses involved in covering the copay for his visits to me—another physician. Thus, I don't know what he has decided. His concern about the financial future of his family is definitely legitimate, but I think another possibility to explain his actions can be considered: he is not sure he actually wants to have the surgery done.

Sure, he has come to me regularly over the past few months for repeated CT scans, as is ordinarily done, to explore the merits of one surgeon versus another, to hear his determination as he looks for a new job, and to assuage his worries regarding his multiple chronic conditions. At the same time, I am also giving him permission to continue in his course of monitoring. At each visit, he says, "I don't think I can have the surgery done now—do you think it is okay if I wait a bit until I am able to get more money together for a nest egg?" And each time I have more or less the same response. No, I cannot make the risk for an aneurysm go away, but, by the same token, the mere presence of a health risk does not obligate the bearer of that risk to try and eliminate it or mitigate it or, in fact, do anything at all to change his present course.

AVOIDING FALSE CERTAINTY
BY THINKING CAREFULLY

This does not mean that Mr. B has resigned himself to pursuing his current course forever. He is carefully thinking about it at every encounter with me, and at every visit he is weighing the risk and benefit. His financial concerns are real, and that is the reason he is comfortable discussing explicitly with me. But the real decision he is making by waiting is not to have surgery, a seemingly obvious point but one often overlooked. Health care decisions are not made at a given point in time but longitudinally, which makes it all the more imperative to avoid false certainty. The only thing certain in the end is that we die; the nature of our death remains to be seen, but on the way there, we should not feel that we must make a particular decision at a given time.

However, there is more to dealing with uncertainty than just avoiding rash decisions. We need to have a strategy in order to approach a future of developments regarding our health of which we cannot be sure. We need to be prepared for whatever might happen in the future. But how do we prepare for future developments in our health when we are not sure what those will be?

TRANSFORMATIVE EXPERIENCES

A category of future experiences has been addressed by the philosopher L. A. Paul in her work *Transformative Experience.*[9] In essence, she asks the question: When life presents important choices, what should one do, especially concerning choices about which one has incomplete information? She lays out the difficulty well: When we face large choices, "we don't know what our lives will be like until we've undergone the new experience, but if we don't undergo the experience, we don't know what we are missing. . . . You know that undergoing the experience will change what it is like for you to live your life, and perhaps even change what it is like to be you, deeply and fundamentally."[10] Sure, you can get advice and testimony from friends and acquaintances about what a change might be like, but Paul points out that such evidence is, of necessity, incomplete. In the end, she says, "we must [weigh] incomplete evidence in the light of our own personal preferences."[11]

How do we weigh, and what criteria should we eventually use to decide? Paul points out that "we only learn what we need to know after we've done it, and we change ourselves in the process of doing it."[12] Thus, she concludes (after making detailed arguments based on numerous disciplines throughout a full-length book of philosophy) that "the best response to this situation is to choose based on whether we want to discover who we'll become."[13]

We can take issue with that last phrase: "discovering who we will become" is not the attitude that we take with our health, because by and large we understand that much of life does involve physical decline.

However, a change in attitude might be in order. Changes in life are a process of discovery, and health-related changes no less so. Thus, as we confront future developments with uncertain information, we should not take at face value the algorithms that we are supposed to follow; instead, we should follow our preferences about the lives that we choose to lead.

12

REVISITING THE BIOMEDICAL PARADIGM

Our health care system adopts superficially novel approaches every few decades. Whether through the deliberate advancement of scientists or clinicians, as a reaction to social change, or through the random flapping of a butterfly's wings, things change—and many people (patients, families, caregivers, ordinary people of all kinds, and even some health care professionals) are not always privy to the discussions underlying such changes or how they might impact our health and health care.

We are currently in the midst of such a change. One ideology is uneasily coexisting with another, and this book is an attempt to bridge ideologies that have been trying to occupy the same space.

One is evidence-based medicine (EBM), as we referred to it in the introduction. The idea behind EBM is that medicine is the application of the best possible scientific evidence to health care options so that patients can make informed decisions. The problems with this view are many, and we have discussed some of them: decisions are not necessarily at the core of what we want from health care; scientific evidence is not all that it is cracked up to be, even at the best of times; and privileging a scientific notion of what evidence is relegates our values and preferences as things to be applied ex post facto, not a priori. One can argue, however, that EBM applies a unifying, if not consistent, intellectual standard to a farrago of diverse practices that has long characterized our doctors and hospitals.

EBM came onto the stage in the 1970s and 1980s (though its roots can be traced to the 1950s and 1960s).[1]

About the same time, however, came new realizations about the individual's role in decision making and that every person should be allowed autonomous decisions, noncoerced. This move toward autonomy, which owed much to realizations from the worst aspects of clinical trials research, emphasized the personhood of the decision maker.[2]

Finally, parallel to this phenomenon, but undoubtedly influenced by it, is the concept of shared decision making, in which we and our doctors deliberate together in order to come to a decision that seems right for us.[3]

As we have seen, these three philosophies do not always see eye to eye. Shared decision making includes a collaborative aspect. The patient is not an independent voice alone but a deliberating mind that interacts with his or her physician. No physician (or other health care provider) means no shared decision making. This doesn't square with autonomy; according to shared decision making, decisions aren't to be made by oneself.

However, autonomy and EBM are not the warmest of partners. If an autonomous individual chooses to do what she desires in the face of the population-based evidence that presumes to speak for her, she acts well according to her lights. But a doctor steeped in the ethos of EBM might not understand her approach. Nor, for that matter, does shared decision making as it is often practiced include a recognition that a shared decision maker can opt out of the sharing.

Every individual is unique. Not merely in the commonplace sense that each person is a slightly different mix of preferences and aspirations, disappointments, accomplishments, pain, and pleasure, but each person has to go through their own process of discovery. You can't replace one person's time line with another or shave off bits of a population until you get down to the level of an individual. One is not reducible to the other. Each of us must make his or her own decisions. Even if we are part of a disadvantaged group and suffer on that basis—encountering barriers that a member of another group might not experience—we must still encounter every day as our own person.

The same message applies to each one of the conditions we have discussed throughout this book. In hypertension, diabetes, chronic pain, arthritis, surgery, and all treatment in general, medicine does less than is often claimed, and, in many cases, does not produce foolproof benefits without harms. What is more, the balance of these benefits and harms cannot be predicted for a given individual.

How do we solve this conundrum? Surely, when a medical condition is diagnosed, doing nothing is not a reasonable choice. What is the point of these diagnoses if they do not point us to potential beneficial treatments?

Let's take a step back. We must consider again, as we have elsewhere in this book, the potential definitions of *health*. To paraphrase a point made by Robert Smith in his blog at the *British Medical Journal*,[4] adopting the definition of the World Health Organization that health is a complete state of wellness would mean that all of us, at some time or another, are more or less unhealthy. We are full of malfunction and mistake, which starts at our birth and does not become less frequent with time—just the opposite, in fact. We say jokingly to each other and our doctors, "Am I falling apart?" but we really know in our heart of hearts that such disintegration is the human condition—the condition of every organism.

To the extent that medicine can diagnose conditions that make a difference to our lives, it is doing us a favor. To the extent that medicine is finding problems that would probably be there anyway, in any life, no favor is being done.

Imagine a spectrum of conditions that medicine can treat—some of them without any importance to us at all, just names of diagnoses that everyone gets and that will not reduce our quality of life or our years lived, and, on the other end of the spectrum, conditions that are of vital importance, not just to life and limb themselves but also to how we live our lives.

Unfortunately, the spectrum is a lot more complicated than that. There are some diseases that can cause increased mortality—that is, a shortened life expectancy—in some people but no problem at all in others (e.g., hypertension). There are others that can alter life for many of those who experience it—rare are those who do not suffer significant consequences (e.g., from stroke). And for still others, there are diseases that are named conditions, which tend not to cause significant problems at all ("thyroid nodule," for instance).[5]

In short, the biomedical paradigm of identifying conditions (diseases) through signs and symptoms, following them up with diagnosis, and pursuing effective treatment is not the only effective path to help. It can even lead to harm. Following the biomedical model[6] means treating the patient like a collection of diseases or a butterfly pinned to an index card in the natural history museum. Such an approach has benefited many people.

While many of the mortality benefits society has enjoyed in the past centuries has, as is well known, not been due to the work of doctors or biomedical scientists, but rather to improvements in public health and hygiene, the health benefits—in mortality and quality of life—due to the biomedical paradigm should not be overlooked. Were it not for a molecular understanding of heart disease, the use of aspirin and other medications would not have significantly reduced mortality. Were it not for antibiotics, there would be many more deaths from bacterial infections. The list goes on.

However, the biomedical paradigm falls short in two big contexts of daily life: first, in our own individual understanding of our health problems, and second, in our ability to navigate for our own interests inside the institutional and societal barriers that restrict our actions.

In our own individual understanding, we do not consider ourselves as collections of diseases or merely a series of diagnoses; in that case, I would be just a forty-two-year-old male with migraines, oculocutaneous albinism, and poor fine-motor coordination. The patient I mention in the chapter on hypertension, Mr. D, would be a sixty-year-old man with high blood pressure, panic disorder, and a history of depression.

But people don't think of themselves in that way. We see ourselves as whole people; our diseases are a part of us but are not constituent of us. This explains a phenomenon that doctors and other health care providers find quite disconcerting: when we, as patients, do not fully follow their directions, whether it's taking medications or changing our lives to fit the dictates of disease-specific guidelines. It's not that we don't think these medical conditions are important, but they do not fully define our actions.

Conversely, if we do not understand ourselves merely as collections of diseases, diagnosing every condition that is wrong with us does not mean that we are thereby more fully empowered to live life, unless we are thereby provided with the tools to improve our symptoms or our life itself.

Thus, the very process in which medical care is often provided does not recognize the circumstances of our individual lives, which are not governed by the principle of find-broken-thing-and-fix-it but most often by make-do-with-what-we-have.

Cataloging diseases through systematic diagnosis does not necessarily lend itself to the improvement of public health, either. The problems of public health—that is, the greatest health challenges faced by the greatest number (in a utilitarian conception)[7] or those faced by the most vulnerable (in a conception of justice based on equal distribution of resources)—are due not to the number of diseases reckoned to affect each individual but to the combination of factors that help determine them.

Many diseases have similar risk factors in common. Many is the time that the resident—doctor-in-training—will remark about a patient that he or she has "all the common stuff" or "the usual stuff," referring to a combination of coronary artery disease, hypertension, diabetes, and high cholesterol, which is indeed common in a lot of people. Except that this combination is actually not just a collection of diseases together but also the fruit, to a large extent, of economic and physical stressors, inequality, unhealthful diet, lack of opportunities for exercise, and other social determinants of health.[8] Speaking of it as a combination of individual diseases misses the point.

So if individual disease finding does not work all the time for individuals or populations, should it be abandoned? What other paradigms are there, and how does the biomedical paradigm fit in with them? Where do we go from here?

One direction I like to take is the "real-life paradigm." While a doctor sees a patient for ten or fifteen minutes at a time (or, in practices with more generous appointment lengths, thirty or sixty minutes), we live the vast majority of our lives outside of the doctor's office and hospital. The disease treatments and tests must fit themselves into our lives, not the other way around. Thus, if a treatment disrupts our routine (whether in school, work, marriage, social interactions, housing, or childrearing), it is less likely to become incorporated into our lives—even if we believe the doctor who is convinced that the medication or other treatment is the right one for us.

Ms. R, a sixty-year-old, professional, African American woman who works in administration at a local university, has chronic migraine headaches that cause her to miss work several times a month. She takes over-the-counter headache medication, containing caffeine, among other things, about ten or twelve days a month, and I have advised her time and again that these migraine medications are not the best thing for her. Why does she keep taking them?

Because they work for her at the moment; she is loath to switch to something else because she has tried things that other doctors have prescribed for her previously and they did not work for her, making her unable to work sufficient days during the month of that trial. So she was out a few days of work because she tried a medication that ended up not being effective for her.

Thus, she has settled on a medication for her migraines that might actually be making them happen more often. Rebound headache is a widely recognized phenomenon that can be associated with taking regular, over-the-counter headache medication on a frequent basis, meaning somewhere around ten times a month. I told her that the frequency with which she is using the over-the-counter headache medications can make them worse, and she understands that, but nonetheless she continues to take these medications at that frequency.

One can guess at various reasons why. Perhaps the medications I recommended for migraine headaches are more expensive than the over-the-counter variety. It could also be that she is reluctant to switch from a treatment that works for her and that the opportunity costs to switching to a new medication—with the trial and error that this process involves—are simply too unrealistic to bear. This reluctance leads people to underconsider possible beneficial alternatives in situations of uncertainty, a phenomenon called *status quo bias*.[9]

However, in this case I have another hypothesis, and it is based on an interaction we have frequently, in which I tell her, time and again, that she has migraines (in my estimation and in the experience of a doctor who has seen a number of patients with migraines and treated them to their satisfaction). She never said the word *migraines*. I was not offended by this; in fact, it happens not infrequently that people do not accept the diagnoses I arrive at. But I thought something might have been going on in this case. She kept referring to her headaches as "regular headaches."

It is true that there is no definitive test to distinguish "migraine" from "tension" from other sorts of headaches. Perhaps for that reason the diagnosis lacks the same "prestige" that others might, not arousing the same fear of perilous consequences. And for that reason, Ms. R might have felt free to treat a migraine like an "ordinary" headache, like a problem that she can deal with on her own terms.

How do we know the difference between the trivial and the serious? How do we know which problems are properly "medicalized"?

That is a difficult question to answer because we do not know in advance what will happen. We cannot absolutely predict which common, everyday symptoms will develop into something serious, nor can we predict which already-diagnosed problems will resolve or remain stable. We can only go by probabilities. In response to this inadequacy, we should take two approaches.

First, since our predictive powers are of necessity limited, I think we should limit, to the extent possible, the worry over future health problems and concentrate on how we feel now. This seems counterintuitive. We are told wherever we turn that we should take care of our health, that preventive health measures can save lives and improve our health in the future, and that ignoring that truth is foolhardy.

I am not denying the importance and usefulness of some such tests, the most useful (the ones I use daily in my practice) being screening tests for colorectal cancer and, possibly, for breast cancer, as well as vaccines against infectious disease and cervical cancer. (Pediatricians and parents of young children are a lot more familiar with preventive measures that can improve children's health.)

So there are individual tests that can improve health in the future. However, I worry that the approach to quality improvement of our health care systems, encouraging approaches to care that increase uptake of such tests, might overemphasize their effectiveness.

If preventive tests might be overemphasized, if we cannot predict the future with great certainty, and if most health problems might resolve, what should we do? What advice should you listen to?

In many cases, the advice about lifestyle changes, diet, and exercise cannot outweigh the social determinants of health that affect our survival, quality of live, and disease symptoms. We can stop smoking, true, but agency is limited by our family members or friends who smoke or advertisements glorifying cigarette use. We can get more exercise, but not if our neighborhood is impossible to walk in. We can improve our diet, depending on what is available at the local store.

Recently, this point about the social determinants of health was lent additional prominence in the public eye via a mistaken column by David Brooks in the *New York Times*, which proposed that poor Americans (by implication, since he did not discuss this phenomenon among upper-income Americans) were distinguished by cultural failure. If only the culture were to be improved in these classes, Brooks implies, they would have improved economic outcomes. [10]

The same implication is leveled daily at those of us with less advantages, less money, and membership in disadvantaged subgroups by doctors and other health care providers. Indeed, in many of the trials of disease treatments based on the biomedical model, such implications are taken to be part and parcel of the way doctors should work and the way the health care system should operate. If only we ate better, we wouldn't be obese. If only we exercised more, our blood pressure wouldn't be high. If only we got out and did more enjoyable activities, we wouldn't be depressed.

Somewhere in between the social determinants of our health, which are very difficult to change, and the interventions promoted by doctors and pharmaceutical companies, which help some of the time but not for everyone and often not without significant harms, are things that we can do to improve our own health that are not part of the medical system or dependent on medical evidence but based on common sense.

Common sense is a dangerous category to have recourse to. It can't be defined. It is prone to error. We can be easily led astray by the mistaken advice of those we trust. But I think it is underrecognized in the maze of health care options that are offered to us like so many expensive items in the window of the jeweler's or tempting options on the menu of the fancy restaurant. Common sense does not necessarily refer to any putative wisdom of crowds, as we know that conventional health wisdom can be wrong. In fact, we know that much of contemporary health care culture is misguided, desiring overtesting and overtreatment. Doctors, insurance companies, and hospitals are to blame for this state of affairs, but certainly part of it is due to our assumption that the consumer—us—is always right and more is certainly better. So if by common sense we mean conventional wisdom, we should certainly not follow it unthinkingly.

On the other hand, if common sense depends on some characteristic of an individual whose decisions should be respected, as is the current trend in health care (going by the name of shared decision making), then common sense is something to be celebrated, the potential savior of ourselves from health care that promises too much, costs too much, and doesn't deliver.

The balance of benefits and harms that characterize potential things that doctors or hospitals do might be unique for each individual. While this uniqueness is particularly fraught in the end-of-life situation, it also exists even in the most seemingly insignificant decisions of everyday life. Common sense means that such everyday decisions should be respected even if they are not a subset of decisions that one is "supposed" to make, even if we do not recognize supposedly incontrovertible benefits.

It is through common sense that a way out of the overmedicalization dilemma might be possible. If we find something that bothers us and we cannot figure out what it is, then—this is so crazy it just might work—we might talk to a health care professional.

But we should not labor under the delusion that we need to see a health care provider regularly if we feel otherwise well. Indeed, there is no strong evidence that—absent health conditions or symptoms—we need to see a doctor at some arbitrarily defined interval.[11]

Even if we have one of the health conditions addressed in this book, it does not automatically follow that we must see the doctor on a predetermined frequency.

We can receive a diagnosis, or set of diagnoses, from a doctor and thereafter pursue care "under our own recognizance"—that is, using those tools that we have developed in the course of ordinary life, observing our own symptoms and figuring out what works for us by trial and error.

I am not counseling you never to rely on doctors' specialized knowledge—that would be irresponsible. I simply mean that in the great majority of cases, medical evidence has not developed to a point where it improves on common strategies for everyday illnesses. In the diagnoses in which medicine has managed spectacular advances (for example, in the treatment of heart disease), mortality improvements have come through taking medications regularly, not through seeing doctors at arbitrarily regular intervals.

Where will common sense fail? When we have urgent medical matters, life-threatening diagnoses, symptoms that we cannot deal with. But health maintenance, as a category, has been significantly overemphasized from a doctor-patient and public health perspective.

The ordinary lumps and bumps of everyday life, the sprained ankles and chronic back pain, can often be left alone. Doing X-rays on chronic pain does not often lead to favorable outcomes.

Tension headaches can also be left alone. So can most upper-respiratory infections.

You know a friend or relative who had a common condition and did not see a physician—that person had some horrible diagnosis and met a terrible fate. These are horrible stories, of course, and should not be discounted. But could anything have been done about that particular situation? The person we know who had a cough that turned out to be cancer—what a terrible tragedy, if there were some way to prevent it. But screening tests for cancer are not pursued without some balance of risks and benefits, and applying them wholesale—especially for the sake of common symptoms that might go away by themselves—is not to be recommended.

There are other examples of so-called normal things that people do, ostensibly for their health, that are not based on good evidence and reflect a naive view of how health care works: if something is wrong, you must (so this assumption goes) take something for it or do something about it. For example, something as simple as taking a daily multivitamin, beloved by many Americans, is not associated with any health benefits, or at least not with any that can be determined from the latest evidence. [12] And getting pictures (images) of back pain does not lead to any advantage for the person getting them, because back pain in itself is not often associated with a major problem.

As we have learned, even treatment of the diseases that are quite common in the community (for example, diabetes) does not necessarily save lives or reduce symptoms if strictly treated with the most advanced pharmacology.

If I were to encapsulate the advice of commonsense self-care, it would be to live your life. See the doctor when things bother you significantly. Don't think you need to see the doctor for every little thing.

But when something does happen, what do we do? We don't have to have recourse to the biomedical paradigm, either—in that case, mistakenly thinking that the diagnose-to-treat-and-cure promises are the only thing that will make us feel better. We should, of course, not abandon modern technology or medicine in all its guises, but we should be judicious about accepting its promises. We should know when the ballyhooed findings of population-based biomedical science are not necessarily going to lead to benefits for us as individuals.

We need to make the jump from health science in populations to a science of the individual, to empirical investigations in health that recognize how different people are unique.

What do I mean by a science of the individual?

Let us take the example of the treatment of blood pressure, which I discussed earlier in this book.

Population science tells us that controlling blood pressure reduces heart attack and stroke. However, any given person deciding whether to take medication for blood pressure cannot know if she will be one of the 125 people who must be treated to prevent one stroke or heart attack or one of the 10 people who are harmed by blood pressure medication. The science of the individual would somehow help us understand which individual patients are likely to be affected by either bad outcome—the heart attack or stroke, on the one hand, and the harm from medication, on the other. [13]

One approach to the science of the individual, from the heady early days of the human genome project, [14] was to posit that each individual's collection of genes is what makes them an individual. This is a reductionist approach to medical science. While the original article is somewhat dated, the vision lives anew in our days due to the precision medicine program, a recent initiative from the National Institutes of Health. [15] President Obama announced this initiative for the first time during his State of the Union address in 2015. The claim in precision medicine is that a reductionist approach to treatment, based on genomics, proteomics, and a greater understanding of the effect of the environment on the individual, can lead to individually tailored treatments.

Two objections to this project make it unlikely that it will be relevant in the near future in bridging population science to individual health. First is that the actual benefits of genomics for patients are surprisingly few, as outlined in an editorial in the *Journal of the American Medical Association*. [16] While treatments for sickle cell disease, for example, have been developed with the techniques grouped under the rubric of "precision medicine," it is unclear whether those techniques will redound in all to the good of patients.

Second is that precision medicine ignores a very real part of the patient's individuality: not the genes (since, after all, genes do not uniquely determine our physiology) but the beliefs and values that go into a patient's physician making—cells, not selves. [17] As individuals, we should have say in the treatments we pursue, or choose not to pursue, in the rubric of shared decision making. Adducing precision medicine as a way to reach the best interests of the individual, without actually including the individual in that process, is a recipe for sinking the precision medicine ship before it has even set sail.

One approach to the science of the individual holds that since there are subpopulations (groups of patients) that differ in risk, there are risk factors that can help determine which category we are likely to fall into as patients—for example, whether we are likely to be helped or hurt by the blood pressure medication.

And a third approach to the individual is to recognize that each person is the driver of his or her own fate and decision making. Science cannot reach to determine the actions of the person because that is not within its realm. Therefore, the science of the individual is just what he or she does, and we should leave off trying to predict risk for any given person. We should embrace the indeterminacy of health futures.

Thus, the most sensible approach to the "science of the individual" for the average person might be to have recourse to one's own "individual science": an empirically based sense of what helps or what does not help in the larger context of what is available for treatment. That is to say, science, based on populations, can give a sense of the possible, but only the individual can decide what might work for herself by understanding how her experiences develop over time, improve, or worsen.

NOTES

INTRODUCTION

1. Wayne Kayton et al., "Depression and Diabetes: A Potentially Lethal Combination," *Journal of General Internal Medicine* 23, no. 10 (2008): 1571–75.

I. CHRONIC PAIN

1. A. D. Furlan et al., "Opioids for Chronic Noncancer Pain: A Meta-analysis of Effectiveness and Side Effects," *Canadian Medical Association Journal* 174, no. 11 (May 2006): 1589–94, PubMed (PMID: 16717269), PubMed Central (PMC1459894).

2. Judy Foreman, *A Nation in Pain: Healing Our Biggest Health Problem* (Oxford: Oxford University Press, 2014).

3. E. D. McNicol, A. Midbari, and E. Eisenberg, "Opioids for Neuropathic Pain," *Cochrane Database of Systematic Reviews*, no. 8 (2013), article no. CD006146, doi:10.1002/14651858.CD006146.pub2.

4. F. Denk, S. B. McMahon, and I. Tracey, "Pain Vulnerability: A Neurobiological Perspective," *Nature Neuroscience* 17, no. 2 (February 2014): 192–200.

5. S. Morley, C. Eccleston, and A. Williams, "Systematic Review and Meta-analysis of Randomized Controlled Trials of Cognitive Behaviour Therapy and Behaviour Therapy for Chronic Pain in Adults, Excluding Headache," *PAIN* 80, no. 1–2 (March 1999): 1–13, PubMed (PMID: 10204712).

6. T. Ojala et al., "The Dominance of Chronic Pain: A Phenomenological Study," *Musculoskeletal Care*, January 15, 2014, doi:10.1002/msc.1066.

7. Thomas Sydenham, *The Works of Thomas Sydenham, MD, on Acute and Chronic Diseases: With Their Histories and Modes of Cure* (Philadelphia: B. & T. Kite, 1809), Research Publications Early American Medical Imprints collection reel 91, no. 1845.

8. C. Eccleston, A. C. Williams, and W. S. Rogers, "Patients' and Professionals' Understandings of the Causes of Chronic Pain: Blame, Responsibility and Identity Protection," *Social Science and Medicine* 45, no. 5 (September 1997): 699–709.

9. Andrew R. Block, Ephrem Fernandez, and Edwin Kremer, eds., *Handbook of Pain Syndromes: Biopsychosocial Perspectives* (New York: Psychology Press, 2013).

10. Furlan et al., "Opioids for Chronic Noncancer Pain," 1589–94.

11. H. L. Fields, "The Doctor's Dilemma: Opiate Analgesics and Chronic Pain," *Neuron* 69, no. 4 (February 2011): 591–94, doi:10.1016/j.neuron.2011.02.001, PubMed (PMID: 21338871), PubMed Central (PMC3073133).

12. Lenore Manderson and Carolyn Smith-Morris, *Chronic Conditions, Fluid States: Chronicity and the Anthropology of Illness* (New Brunswick, NJ: Rutgers University Press, 2010).

13. Lewis S. Nelson, David N. Juurlink, and Jeanmarie Perrone, "Addressing the Opioid Epidemic," *Journal of the American Medical Association* 314, no. 14 (2015): 1453–54.

14. Michael Von Korff et al., "Long-Term Opioid Therapy Reconsidered," *Annals of Internal Medicine* 155, no. 5 (September 11): 325–28.

15. Centers for Disease Control and Prevention, *Wide-Ranging Online Data for Epidemiologic Research (WONDER)*, last reviewed September 15, 2015, http://wonder.cdc.gov/mortsql.html.

16. G. L. Engel, "The Need for a New Medical Model: A Challenge for Biomedicine," *Science* 196, no. 4286 (April 1977): 129–36, doi:10.1126/science.847460.

17. Abraham Verghese and Ralph I. Horwitz, "In Praise of the Physical Examination," *British Medical Journal* 339 (2009): b5448, doi:10.1136/bmj.b5448.

18. B. B. Dean et al., "Effectiveness of Proton Pump Inhibitors in Nonerosive Reflux Disease" (review), *Clinical Gastroenterology and Hepatology* 2, no. 8 (August 2004): 656–64, PubMed (PMID: 15290657).

19. G. P. Gui et al., "Is Cholecystectomy Effective Treatment for Symptomatic Gallstones? Clinical Outcome after Long-Term Follow-Up" (review), *Annals of the Royal College of Surgeons of England* 80, no. 1 (January 1998): 25–32, PubMed (PMID: 9579123), PubMed Central (PMC2502763).

2. COMMON CONDITIONS

1. Susan Okie, "A Flood of Opiates, a Rising Tide of Deaths," *New England Journal of Medicine* 363 (2010): 1981–85, doi:10.1056/NEJMp1011512.

2. M. A. Weber et al., "Clinical Practice Guidelines for the Management of Hypertension in the Community: A Statement by the American Society of Hypertension and the International Society of Hypertension," *Journal of Clinical Hypertension* 16, no. 1 (January 2014): 14–26, doi:10.1111/jch.12237, PubMed (PMID: 24341872).

3. R. P. Silva-Néto, K. J. Almeida, and S. N. Bernardino, "Analysis of the Duration of Migraine Prophylaxis," *Journal of the Neurological Sciences* 337, no. 1–2 (February 2014): 38–41, doi:10.1016/j.jns.2013.11.013, PubMed (PMID: 24308946).

4. S. V. Srinivas, R. A. Deyo, and Z. D. Berger, "Application of 'Less Is More' to Low Back Pain," *Archives of Internal Medicine* 172, no. 13 (July 2012): 1016–20, doi:10.1001/archinternmed.2012.1838.

5. Z. D. Berger et al., "Characteristics and Experiences of Patients with Localized Prostate Cancer Who Left an Active Surveillance Program," *Patient* 7, no. 4 (2014): 427–36, doi:10.1007/s40271-014-0066-z, PubMed (PMID: 24920082), PubMed Central (PMC4332784).

6. Berger et al., "Characteristics and Experiences of Patients with Localized Prostate Cancer."

7. S. J. Bielinski et al., "Preemptive Genotyping for Personalized Medicine: Design of the Right Drug, Right Dose, Right Time—Using Genomic Data to Individualize Treatment Protocol," *Mayo Clinic Proceedings* 89, no. 1 (January 2014): 25–33, doi:10.1016/j.mayocp.2013.10.021, PubMed (PMID: 24388019), PubMed Central (PMC3932754).

3. POVERTY

1. Centers for Disease Control and Prevention, "Get Smart for Healthcare," last updated September 15, 2015, www.cdc.gov/getsmart/healthcare/.

2. C. van Walraven and C. D. Naylor, "Do We Know What Inappropriate Laboratory Utilization Is? A Systematic Review of Laboratory Clinical Audits," *Journal of the American Medical Association* 280 (1998): 550–58.

3. Vijay M. Rao and David C. Levin, "The Overuse of Diagnostic Imaging and the Choosing Wisely Initiative," *Annals of Internal Medicine* 157, no. 8 (2012): 574–76.

4. Dennis P. Andrulis, "Access to Care Is the Centerpiece in the Elimination of Socioeconomic Disparities in Health," *Annals of Internal Medicine* 129, no. 5 (September 1998): 412–16, doi:10.7326/0003-4819-129-5-199809010-00012.

5. Frank R. Lichtenberg, "The Effects of Medicare on Health Care Utilization and Outcomes," *Forum for Health Economics and Policy* 5, no. 1 (January 2002), doi:10.2202/1558-9544.1028.

6. Deborah Grady and Rita F. Redberg, "Less Is More: How Less Health Care Can Result in Better Health," *Archives of Internal Medicine* 170, no. 9 (2010): 749–50.

7. D. Korenstein et al., "Overuse of Health Care Services in the United States: An Understudied Problem," *Archives of Internal Medicine* 172, no. 2 (2012): 171–78, doi:10.1001/archinternmed.2011.772.

8. Anahad O'Connor, "New York Attorney General Targets Supplements at Major Retailers," *Well* (blog), *New York Times*, February 3, 2015, http://well. blogs.nytimes.com/2015/02/03/new-york-attorney-general-targets-supplements-at-major-retailers.

9. J. T. Edelson et al., "Long-Term Cost-Effectiveness of Various Initial Monotherapies for Mild to Moderate Hypertension," *Journal of the American Medical Association* 263, no. 3 (1990): 407–13, doi:10.1001/jama.1990.034 40030094028.

10. W. B. Borden, Y. P. Chiang, and R. Kronick, "Bringing Patient-Centered Outcomes Research to Life" (review), *Value Health* 18, no. 4 (June 2015): 355–57, doi:10.1016/j.jval.2015.01.010, PubMed (PMID: 26091588).

11. Methodology Committee of the Patient-Centered Outcomes Research Institute (PCORI), "Methodological Standards and Patient-Centeredness in Comparative Effectiveness Research: The PCORI Perspective," *Journal of the American Medical Association* 307, no. 15 (2012): 1636–40.

12. Ta-Nehisi Coates, "The Case for Reparations," *Atlantic*, June 2014, www. theatlantic.com/magazine/archive/2014/06/the-case-for-reparations/361631/.

13. Karen Davis et al., *Mirror, Mirror on the Wall: How the Performance of the U.S. Health Care System Compares Internationally: 2014 Update* (New York: Commonwealth Fund, 2014), accessed September 21, 2015, www. commonwealthfund.org/~/media/files/publications/fund-report/2014/jun/1755_ davis_mirror_mirror_2014.pdf.

14. "Reflections on Variations," *The Dartmouth Atlas of Health Care*, last updated 2015, accessed September 21, 2015, www.dartmouthatlas.org/ keyissues/issue.aspx?con=1338.

15. "Bariatric Surgery per 100,000 Medicare Enrollees: Year: 2007–11; Region Level: HRR," *The Dartmouth Atlas of Health Care*, accessed September 21, 2015, www.dartmouthatlas.org/data/map.aspx?ind=299&tf=29&loct=3&extent= -14071323.410590487%202305693.8872850095%20-7398676.589409513%20

6806306.112714991%2C-14071323.410590487%202110015.09487501%20-7398676.589409513%207001984.90512499.

16. K. E. Joynt, E. J. Orav, and A. K. Jha, "The Association between Hospital Volume and Processes, Outcomes, and Costs of Care for Congestive Heart Failure," *Annals of Internal Medicine* 154 (2011): 94–102, doi:10.7326/0003-4819-154-2-201101180-00008.

17. Joseph J. Doyle et al., "Measuring Returns to Hospital Care: Evidence from Ambulance Referral Patterns," *Journal of Political Economy* 123, no. 1 (2015): 170–214.

18. P. S. Hussey, S. Wertheimer, and A. Mehrotra, "The Association between Health Care Quality and Cost: A Systematic Review," *Annals of Internal Medicine* 158 (2013): 27–34, doi:10.7326/0003-4819-158-1-201301010-00006.

19. Uwe E. Reinhardt, "Waste vs. Value in American Health Care," *Economix* (blog), *New York Times*, September 13, 2013, accessed September 21, 2015, http://economix.blogs.nytimes.com/2013/09/13/waste-vs-value-in-american-health-care/.

20. Centers for Medicare and Medicaid Services, Hospital Compare, last modified December 4, 2015, www.cms.gov/medicare/quality-initiatives-patient-assessment-instruments/hospitalqualityinits/hospitalcompare.html.

21. Medicare.gov, Physician Compare, www.medicare.gov/physiciancompare/search.html.

22. Lena Groeger et al., "Dollars for Docs: How Industry Dollars Reach Your Doctors," *Pro Publica*, updated July 1, 2015, https://projects.propublica.org/docdollars/.

4. DEPRESSION

1. Norbert Stefan et al., "Metabolically Healthy Obesity: Epidemiology, Mechanisms, and Clinical Implications," *Lancet: Diabetes and Endocrinology* 1, no. 2 (2013): 152–62.

2. See, for example, John Bowlby, *Loss: Sadness and Depression*, Attachment and Loss 3 (New York: Basic Books, 1980).

3. Annemarie Moll, *The Logic of Care: Health and the Problem of Patient Choice* (London and New York: Routledge, 2008).

4. Michael Polanyi and Amartya Sen, *The Tacit Dimension* (New York: Doubleday, 1967).

5. American Psychiatric Association, *Diagnostic and Statistical Manual of Mental Disorders*, 5th ed. (*DSM-5®*) (Washington, DC: American Psychiatric Publishing, 2013).

6. S. Dimidjian et al., "Randomized Trial of Behavioral Activation, Cognitive Therapy, and Antidepressant Medication in the Acute Treatment of Adults with Major Depression," *Journal of Consulting and Clinical Psychology* 74, no. 4 (August 2006): 658–70, doi:10.1037/0022-006X.74.4.658.

7. F. K. Vergunst et al., "Longitudinal Course of Symptom Severity and Fluctuation in Patients with Treatment-Resistant Unipolar and Bipolar Depression," *Psychiatry Research* 207, no. 3 (May 2013): 143–49, doi:10.1016/j.psychres.2013.03.022, PubMed (PMID: 23601791).

8. Colleen L. Barry and Haiden A. Huskamp, "Moving beyond Parity— Mental Health and Addiction Care under the ACA," *New England Journal of Medicine* 365 (September 2011): 973–75, doi:10.1056/NEJMp1108649.

9. J. Angst and K. Merikangas, "The Depressive Spectrum: Diagnostic Classification and Course," *Journal of Affective Disorders* 45, nos. 1–2 (August 1997): 31–39, discussion 39–40, PubMed (PMID: 9268773).

10. Zachary Berger, *Talking to Your Doctor: A Patient's Guide to Communication in the Exam Room and Beyond* (Lanham, MD: Rowman & Littlefield, 2013).

11. Gary Schwitzer, "'Potential Biomarker That Could Predict'?—Caveats about Psychiatric Brain Imaging and Blogging about It," HealthNewsReview.org, January 20, 2015, www.healthnewsreview.org/2015/01/potential-biomarker-that-could-predict-caveats-about-psychiatric-brain-imaging-blogging-about-it/.

12. E. A. O'Connor et al., "Screening for Depression in Adult Patients in Primary Care Settings: A Systematic Evidence Review," *Annals of Internal Medicine* 151 (2009): 793–803, doi:10.7326/0003-4819-151-11-200912010-0.

13. Kathryn Rost et al., "Improving Depression Outcomes in Community Primary Care Practice," *Journal of General Internal Medicine* 16, no. 3 (2001): 143–49.

14. *Stanford Encyclopedia of Philosophy*, s.v. "Virtue Ethics," by Rosalind Hursthouse, last revised March 8, 2012, http://plato.stanford.edu/entries/ethics-virtue/.

15. Richard Friedman, "When All Else Fails, Blaming the Patient Comes Next," *New York Times*, October 20, 2008, www.nytimes.com/2008/10/21/health/21mind.html.

16. M. E. Farmer et al., "Physical Activity and Depressive Symptoms: The NHANES I Epidemiologic Follow-Up Study," *American Journal of Epidemiology* 128, no. 6 (December 1988): 1340–51, PubMed (PMID: 3264110).

5. HIGH BLOOD PRESSURE

1. Brent M. Egan, Yumin Zhao, and R. Neal Axon, "US Trends in Prevalence, Awareness, Treatment, and Control of Hypertension, 1988–2008," *Journal of the American Medical Association* 303, no. 20 (May 2010): 2043–50, doi:10.1001/jama.2010.650.

2. Egan, Zhao, and Axon, "US Trends in Prevalence."

3. J. T. Wright, "The Benefits of Detecting and Treating Mild Hypertension: What We Know, and What We Need to Learn," *Annals of Internal Medicine* 162 (2015): 233–34, doi:10.7326/M14-2836.

4. P. K. Whelton, "The Elusiveness of Population-Wide High Blood Pressure Control," *Annual Review of Public Health* 36 (March 2015): 109–30, doi:10.1146/annurev-publhealth-031914-122949, PubMed (PMID: 25594330).

5. Yendelela Cuffee et al., "Psychosocial Risk Factors for Hypertension: An Update of the Literature," *Current Hypertension Reports* 16, no. 10 (October 2014): 1–11, doi:10.1007/s11906-014-0483-3, PubMed (PMID: 25139781), PubMed Central (PMC4163921).

6. Cuffee et al., "Psychosocial Risk Factors for Hypertension," 1–11.

7. Axel Bauer, "'Die Medicin ist eine sociale Wissenschaft'—Rudolf Virchow (1821–1902) als Pathologe, Politiker, Publizist," *GMS Medizin—Bibliothek—Information* 5, no. 1 (2005): Doc01.

8. M. A. Weber et al., "Clinical Practice Guidelines for the Management of Hypertension in the Community: A Statement by the American Society of Hypertension and the International Society of Hypertension," *Journal of Clinical Hypertension* 16, no. 1 (January 2014): 14–26, doi:10.1111/jch.12237, PubMed (PMID: 24341872).

9. M. A. Piper et al., "Diagnostic and Predictive Accuracy of Blood Pressure Screening Methods with Consideration of Rescreening Intervals: A Systematic Review for the U.S. Preventive Services Task Force," *Annals of Internal Medicine* 162 (2015): 192–204, doi:10.7326/M14-1539.

10. SPRINT Research Group, "A Randomized Trial of Intensive versus Standard Blood-Pressure Control," *New England Journal of Medicine* 373, no. 22 (November 2015): 2103–16, doi:10.1056/NEJMoa1511939, PubMed (PMID: 26551272).

6. DIABETES

1. Richard Lehman, "Richard Lehman's Journal Review—16 February 2015," *BMJ Blogs, British Medical Journal*, February 16, 2015, http://blogs.bmj.com/bmj/2015/02/16/richard-lehmans-journal-review-16-february-2015/.

2. L. I. Rand and F. L. Ferris III, "Long-Term Contributions from the Diabetes Control and Complications Trial Cohort," *JAMA Ophthalmology*, August 13, 2015, doi:10.1001/jamaophthalmol.2015.2735.

3. S. Inzucchi and S Majumdar, "Glycemic Targets: What Is the Evidence?" (review), *Medical Clinics of North America* 99, no. 1 (January 2015): 47–67, doi:10.1016/j.mcna.2014.08.018. Erratum: *Medical Clinics of North America* 99, no. 2 (March 2015): xix.

4. Kasia J. Lipska et al., "Potential Overtreatment of Diabetes Mellitus in Older Adults with Tight Glycemic Control," *JAMA Internal Medicine* 175, no. 3 (2015): 356–62.

5. Zackary Berger and Dave deBronkart, "'Precision Medicine' Needs Patient Partnership," *BMJ Blogs, BMJ*, March 20, 2015, http://blogs.bmj.com/bmj/2015/03/20/zackary-berger-and-dave-debronkart-precision-medicine-needs-patient-partnership/.

6. R. Rubin, "Precision Medicine: The Future or Simply Politics?" *Journal of the American Medical Association* 313, no. 11 (2015): 1089–91, doi:10.1001/jama.2015.0957.

7. Ronald Bayer and Sandro Galea, "Public Health in the Precision-Medicine Era," *New England Journal of Medicine* 373 (August 2015): 499–501, doi:10.1056/NEJMp1506241.

8. N. E. Adler and A. A. Prather, "Risk for Type 2 Diabetes Mellitus: Person, Place, and Precision Prevention," *JAMA Internal Medicine* 175, no. 8 (August 2015): 1321–22, doi:10.1001/jamainternmed.2015.2701.

9. Allan Donner, "A Bayesian Approach to the Interpretation of Subgroup Results in Clinical Trials," *Journal of Chronic Diseases* 35, no. 6 (1982): 429–35.

10. O. Etzion and M. G. Ghany, "A Cure for the High Cost of Hepatitis C Virus Treatment," *Annals of Internal Medicine* 162 (2015): 660–61, doi:10.7326/M15-0674.

11. D. Y. Graham et al., "Effect of Treatment of *Helicobacter pylori* Infection on the Long-Term Recurrence of Gastric or Duodenal Ulcer: A Randomized, Controlled Study," *Annals of Internal Medicine* 116, no. 9 (1992): 705–8, doi:10.7326/0003-4819-116-9-705.

12. D. Y. Graham, Y.-C. Lee, and M.-S. Wu, "Rational *Helicobacter pylori* Therapy: Evidence-Based Medicine Rather Than Medicine-Based Evidence," *Clinical Gastroenterology and Hepatology* 12, no. 2 (February 2014):

177–86.e3, discussion e12–e13, doi:10.1016/j.cgh.2013.05.028, PubMed (PMID: 23751282), PubMed Central (PMC3830667).

7. ARTHRITIS

1. H. C. Wijeysundera and D. T. Ko, "Does Percutaneous Coronary Intervention Reduce Mortality in Patients with Stable Chronic Angina: Are We Talking about Apples and Oranges?" *Circulation: Cardiovascular Quality Outcomes* 2, no. 2 (March 2009): 123–26, doi:10.1161/CIRCOUTCOMES.108.834853, PubMed (PMID: 20031824).

2. Sofia de Achaval et al., "Patients' Expectations about Total Knee Arthroplasty Outcomes," Supplement, *Health Expectations*, no. 4 (February 2015), doi:10.1111/hex.12350.

3. A. D. Beswick et al., "What Proportion of Patients Report Long-Term Pain after Total Hip or Knee Replacement for Osteoarthritis? A Systematic Review of Prospective Studies in Unselected Patients," *BMJ Open* 2, no. 1 (February 2012): e000435, doi:10.1136/bmjopen-2011-000435.

4. Michelle T. Buckius et al., "Changing Epidemiology of Acute Appendicitis in the United States: Study Period 1993–2008," *Journal of Surgical Research* 175, no. 2 (2012): 185–90.

5. David R. Flum, "Acute Appendicitis—Appendectomy or the 'Antibiotics First' Strategy," *New England Journal of Medicine* 372, no. 20 (2015): 1937–43.

6. Marian F. MacDorman, Fay Menacker, and Eugene Declercq, "Cesarean Birth in the United States: Epidemiology, Trends, and Outcomes," *Clinics in Perinatology* 35, no. 2 (2008): 293–307.

7. A. T. Chien and M. B. Rosenthal, "Waste Not, Want Not: Promoting Efficient Use of Health Care Resources," *Annals of Internal Medicine* 158 (2013): 67–68, doi:10.7326/0003-4819-158-1-201301010-00014.

8. Zackary Berger, *Talking to Your Doctor: A Patient's Guide to Communication in the Exam Room and Beyond* (Lanham, MD: Rowman & Littlefield, 2013).

9. Peter Ubel, *Critical Decisions: How You and Your Doctor Can Make the Right Medical Choices Together* (New York: HarperCollins, 2012).

10. E. Roddy, W. Zhang, and M. Doherty, "Aerobic Walking or Strengthening Exercise for Osteoarthritis of the Knee? A Systematic Review," *Annals Rheumatic Diseases* 64, no. 4 (April 2005): 544–48, PubMed (PMID: 15769914), PubMed Central (PMC1755453).

8. SURGERY

1. Amos Tversky and Daniel Kahneman, "The Framing of Decisions and the Psychology of Choice," *Science* 211, no. 4481 (1981): 453–58.

2. Peter Ubel, *Critical Decisions: How You and Your Doctor Can Make the Right Medical Choices Together* (New York: HarperCollins, 2012).

3. Medicare.gov, Physician Compare, www.medicare.gov/physician compare/search.html.

4. A. D. Beswick et al., "What Proportion of Patients Report Long-Term Pain after Total Hip or Knee Replacement for Osteoarthritis? A Systematic Review of Prospective Studies in Unselected Patients," *BMJ Open* 2, no. 1 (February 2012): e000435, doi:10.1136/bmjopen-2011-000435.

5. Bradley N. Reames et al., "Hospital Volume and Operative Mortality in the Modern Era," *Annals of Surgery* 260, no. 2 (August 2014): 244–51, doi:10.1097/SLA.0000000000000375.

9. HOW GOOD CAN GUIDELINES BE?

1. A. J. Barsky, "Hidden Reasons Some Patients Visit Doctors," *Annals of Internal Medicine* 94 (1981): 492–98, doi:10.7326/0003-4819-94-4-492.

2. Sherrie H. Kaplan et al., "Patient and Visit Characteristics Related to Physicians' Participatory Decision-Making Style: Results from the Medical Outcomes Study," *Medical Care* 33, no. 12 (December 1995): 1176–87, www.jstor.org/stable/3766817.

3. H. C. Van Spall et al., "Eligibility Criteria of Randomized Controlled Trials Published in High-Impact General Medical Journals: A Systematic Sampling Review," *Journal of the American Medical Association* 297, no. 11 (2007): 1233–40, doi:10.1001/jama.297.11.1233.

4. A Boivin et al., "Patient and Public Involvement in Clinical Guidelines: International Experiences and Future Perspectives," *Quality and Safety Health Care* 19, no. 5 (October 2010): e22, doi:10.1136/qshc.2009.034835, PubMed (PMID: 20427302).

5. A. M. Stiggelbout, A. H. Pieterse, and J. C. De Haes, "Shared Decision Making: Concepts, Evidence, and Practice," *Patient Education and Counseling* 90, no. 10 (October 2015): 1172–79, doi:10.1016/j.pec.2015.06.022, PubMed (PMID: 26215573).

6. Neil J. Stone et al., "2013 ACC/AHA Guideline on the Treatment of Blood Cholesterol to Reduce Atherosclerotic Cardiovascular Risk in Adults,"

Journal of the American College of Cardiologists 63, no. 25_PA (July 2014): 2889–934, doi:10.1016/j.jacc.2013.11.002.

7. http://www.whosmydoctor.com/styled-3/styled-15/styled-51/Bias.html#. VpV8BfkrIdU.

8. J. Concato, N. Shah, and R. I. Horwitz, "Randomized, Controlled Trials, Observational Studies, and the Hierarchy of Research Designs," *New England Journal of Medicine* 342, no. 25 (June 2000): 1887–92, PubMed (PMID: 10861325), PubMed Central (PMC1557642).

9. L. Bookstein et al., "Day-to-Day Variability of Serum Cholesterol, Trigly-ceride, and High-Density Lipoprotein Cholesterol Levels," *Archives of Internal Medicine* 150, no. 8 (August 1990): 1653–57, doi:10.1001/archinte.1990.0004 0031653012.

10. N. Donner-Banzhoff and A. Sönnichsen, "Strategies for Prescribing Sta-tins," *British Medical Journal* 336, no. 7639 (February 2008): 288–89, doi:10.1136/bmj.39387.573947.80, PubMed (PMID: 18258935), PubMed Cen-tral (PMC2234555).

11. P. M. Ridker and N. R. Cook, "Comparing Cardiovascular Risk Predic-tion Scores," *Annals of Internal Medicine* 162 (2015): 313–14, doi:10.7326/ M14-2820.

12. Ezekiel J. Emanuel and Linda L. Emanuel, "Four Models of the Physi-cian-Patient Relationship," *Journal of the American Medical Association* 267, no. 16 (1992): 2221–26.

13. American College of Cardiology and American Heart Association, ASCVD Risk Estimator, 2014, http://tools.acc.org/ASCVD-Risk-Estimator/.

14. John D. Abramson and Rita F. Redberg, "Don't Give More Patients Sta-tins," *New York Times*, November 13, 2013.

15. Fangjian Guo et al., "Trends in Prevalence, Awareness, Management, and Control of Hypertension among United States Adults, 1999 to 2010," *Journal of the American College of Cardiology* 60, no. 7 (2012): 599–606, doi:10.1016/ j.jacc.2012.04.026.

16. S. S. Martin and R. S. Blumenthal, "Concepts and Controversies: The 2013 American College of Cardiology/American Heart Association Risk Assess-ment and Cholesterol Treatment Guidelines," *Annals of Internal Medicine* 160 (2014): 356–58, doi:10.7326/M13-2805.

10. IS HALF OF ALL RESEARCH WRONG?

1. Patient-Centered Outcomes Research Institute, "Research We Support," last updated October 20, 2015, www.pcori.org/research-results/research-we-support.

2. See, among others, Jordan Ellenberg, *How Not to Be Wrong: The Power of Mathematical Thinking* (New York: Penguin, 2014), and Nate Silver, *The Signal and the Noise: Why So Many Predictions Fail—but Some Don't* (New York: Penguin, 2012).

3. John P. A. Ioannidis, "Why Most Published Research Findings Are False," *Chance* 18, no. 4 (2005): 40–47.

4. Leah R. Jager and Jeffrey T. Leek, "An Estimate of the Science-Wise False Discovery Rate and Application to the Top Medical Literature," *Biostatistics* 15, no. 1 (2014): 1–12.

5. Kirstin Borgerson, "Valuing Evidence: Bias and the Evidence Hierarchy of Evidence-Based Medicine," *Perspectives in Biology and Medicine* 52, no. 2 (2009): 218–33.

6. Khalid Khan et al., *Systematic Reviews to Support Evidence-Based Medicine*, 2nd ed. (Boca Raton, FL, and London: CRC Press, 2011).

7. Thomas Lumley, "Network Meta-analysis for Indirect Treatment Comparisons," *Statistics in Medicine* 21, no. 16 (2002): 2313–24.

11. AVOIDING FALSE CERTAINTY AND APPROACHING FUTURE EXPERIENCES

1. M. E. Hellemons et al., "Validity of Biomarkers Predicting Onset or Progression of Nephropathy in Patients with Type 2 Diabetes: A Systematic Review," *Diabetic Medicine* 29 (2012): 567–77, doi:10.1111/j.1464-5491.2011.03437.x.

2. National Institute of Diabetes and Digestive and Kidney Diseases, *The A1C Test and Diabetes*, NIH Publication 14-7816 (March 2014), under "What A1C target should people have?" www.niddk.nih.gov/health-information/health-topics/diagnostic-tests/a1c-test-diabetes/Pages/index.aspx#15.

3. Dario Giugliano et al., "Setting the Hemoglobin A1C Target in Type 2 Diabetes: A Priori, A Posteriori, or Neither?" *Endocrine* 50, no. 1 (2015): 56–60.

4. William Samuelson and Richard Zeckhauser, "Status Quo Bias in Decision Making," *Journal of Risk and Uncertainty* 1, no. 1 (1988): 7–59.

5. Annmarie Moll, *The Logic of Care: Health and the Problem of Patient Choice* (London and New York: Routledge, 2008).

6. Kim L. Bennell et al., "Effect of Physical Therapy on Pain and Function in Patients with Hip Osteoarthritis: A Randomized Clinical Trial," *Journal of the American Medical Association* 311, no. 19 (2014): 1987–97.

7. Peter Ubel, *Critical Decisions: How You and Your Doctor Can Make the Right Medical Choices Together* (New York: HarperCollins, 2012).

8. Jessica Bylander, "Civil Unrest, Police Use of Force, and the Public's Health," *Health Affairs* 34, no. 8 (2015): 1264–68.

9. Laurie Ann Paul, *Transformative Experience* (Oxford: Oxford University Press, 2014).

10. Paul, *Transformative Experience*, 3.

11. Paul, *Transformative Experience*, 3.

12. Paul, *Transformative Experience*, 4.

13. Paul, *Transformative Experience*, 4.

12. REVISITING THE BIOMEDICAL PARADIGM

1. Stefan Timmermans and Emily S. Kolker, "Evidence-Based Medicine and the Reconfiguration of Medical Knowledge," in "Health and Health Care in the United States: Origins and Dynamics," extra issue, *Journal of Health and Social Behavior* 45 (2004): 177–93.

2. Paul Root Wolpe, "The Triumph of Autonomy in American Bioethics: A Sociological View," in *Bioethics and Society: Constructing the Ethical Enterprise*, ed. Raymond G. De Vries and Janardan Subedi (Upper Saddle River, NJ: Prentice Hall, 1998), 38–59.

3. Adrian Edwards and Glyn Elwyn, *Shared Decision-Making in Health Care: Achieving Evidence-Based Patient Choice* (Oxford: Oxford University Press, 2009).

4. Richard Smith, "The End of Disease and the Beginning of Health," *BMJ Blogs*, *British Medical Journal*, July 8, 2008, http://blogs.bmj.com/bmj/2008/07/08/richard-smith-the-end-of-disease-and-the-beginning-of-health/.

5. Anne R. Cappola and Susan J. Mandel, "Improving the Long-Term Management of Benign Thyroid Nodules," *Journal of the American Medical Association* 313, no. 9 (2015): 903–4.

6. G. L. Engel, "The Need for a New Medical Model: A Challenge for Biomedicine," *Science* 196, no. 4286 (April 1977): 129–36, doi:10.1126/science.847460.

7. Marc J. Roberts and Michael R. Reich, "Ethical Analysis in Public Health," *Lancet* 359, no. 9311 (2002): 1055–59.

8. Richard G. Wilkinson and Michael Gideon Marmot, *Social Determinants of Health: The Solid Facts*, 2nd ed. (Copenhagen: World Health Organization, Regional Office for Europe, 2003).

9. Donald A. Redelmeier and Eldar Shafir, "Medical Decision Making in Situations That Offer Multiple Alternatives," *Journal of the American Medical Association* 273, no. 4 (1995): 302–5.

10. David Brooks, "The Nature of Poverty," *New York Times*, May 1, 2015, www.nytimes.com/2015/05/01/opinion/david-brooks-the-nature-of-poverty.html.

11. Society of General Internal Medicine, "Don't Perform Routine General Health Checks for Asymptomatic Adults," Choosing Wisely, September 12, 2013, www.choosingwisely.org/clinician-lists/society-general-internal-medicine-general-health-checks-for-asymptomatic-adults/.

12. V. A. Moyer and the U.S. Preventive Services Task Force, "Vitamin, Mineral, and Multivitamin Supplements for the Primary Prevention of Cardiovascular Disease and Cancer: U.S. Preventive Services Task Force Recommendation Statement," *Annals of Internal Medicine* 160 (2014): 558–64, doi:10.7326/M14-0198.

13. James McCormack, "Blood Pressure Medicines for Five Years to Prevent Death, Heart Attacks, and Strokes," NNT, July 21, 2014, www.thennt.com/nnt/anti-hypertensives-to-prevent-death-heart-attacks-and-strokes/.

14. B. Childs, C. Weiner, and D. Valle, "A Science of the Individual: Implications for a Medical School Curriculum," *Annual Review of Genomics and Human Genetics* 6 (2005): 313–30.

15. National Institutes of Health, "Precision Medicine Initiative Cohort Program," www.nih.gov/precisionmedicine/.

16. M. J. Khoury and J. P. Evans, "A Public Health Perspective on a National Precision Medicine Cohort: Balancing Long-Term Knowledge Generation with Early Health Benefit," *Journal of the American Medical Association* 313, no. 21 (2015): 2117–18, doi:10.1001/jama.2015.3382.

17. Zackary Berger and Dave deBronkart, "'Precision Medicine' Needs Patient Partnership," *BMJ Blogs*, *British Medical Journal*, March 20, 2015, http://blogs.bmj.com/bmj/2015/03/20/zackary-berger-and-dave-debronkart-precision-medicine-needs-patient-partnership/.

BIBLIOGRAPHY

Achaval, Sofia de, Michael A. Kallen, Benjamin Amick, Glen Landon, Sherwin Siff, David Edelstein, Hong Zhang, and Maria E. Suarez-Almazor. "Patients' Expectations about Total Knee Arthroplasty Outcomes." Supplement, *Health Expectations*, no. 4 (February 2015). doi:10.1111/hex.12350.

Adler, N. E., and A. A. Prather. "Risk for Type 2 Diabetes Mellitus: Person, Place, and Precision Prevention." *JAMA Internal Medicine* 175, no. 8 (August 2015): 1321–22. doi:10.1001/jamainternmed.2015.2701.

American Psychiatric Association. *Diagnostic and Statistical Manual of Mental Disorders*. 5th ed. (*DSM-5®*). Washington, DC: American Psychiatric Publishing, 2013.

Andrulis, Dennis P. "Access to Care Is the Centerpiece in the Elimination of Socioeconomic Disparities in Health." *Annals of Internal Medicine* 129, no. 5 (September 1998): 412–16. doi:10.7326/0003-4819-129-5-199809010-00012.

Angst, J., and K. Merikangas. "The Depressive Spectrum: Diagnostic Classification and Course." *Journal of Affective Disorders* 45, nos. 1–2 (August 1997): 31–39, discussion 39–40. PubMed (PMID: 9268773).

Barry, Colleen L., and Haiden A. Huskamp. "Moving beyond Parity—Mental Health and Addiction Care under the ACA." *New England Journal of Medicine* 365 (September 2011): 973–75. doi:10.1056/NEJMp1108649.

Barsky, A. J. "Hidden Reasons Some Patients Visit Doctors." *Annals of Internal Medicine* 94 (1981): 492–98. doi:10.7326/0003-4819-94-4-492.

Bauer, Axel. "'Die Medicin ist eine sociale Wissenschaft'—Rudolf Virchow (1821–1902) als Pathologe, Politiker, Publizist." *GMS Medizin—Bibliothek—Information* 5, no. 1 (2005).

Bayer, Ronald, and Sandro Galea. "Public Health in the Precision-Medicine Era." *New England Journal of Medicine* 373 (August 2015): 499–501. doi:10.1056/NEJMp1506241.

Bennell, K. L., T. Egerton, J. Martin, J. H. Abbott, B. Metcalf, F. McManus, K. Sims, et al. "Effect of Physical Therapy on Pain and Function in Patients with Hip Osteoarthritis: A Randomized Clinical Trial." *Journal of the American Medical Association* 311, no. 19 (2014): 1987–97.

Berger, Zackary. *Talking to Your Doctor: A Patient's Guide to Communication in the Exam Room and Beyond*. Lanham, MD: Rowman & Littlefield, 2013.

Berger, Z. D., J. C. Yeh, H. B. Carter, and C. E. Pollack. "Characteristics and Experiences of Patients with Localized Prostate Cancer Who Left an Active Surveillance Program." *Patient* 7, no. 4 (2014): 427–36. doi:10.1007/s40271-014-0066-z. PubMed (PMID: 24920082). PubMed Central (PMC4332784).

Beswick, A. D., V. Wylde, R. Gooberman-Hill, A. Blom, and P. Dieppe. "What Proportion of Patients Report Long-Term Pain after Total Hip or Knee Replacement for Osteoarthritis?

A Systematic Review of Prospective Studies in Unselected Patients." *BMJ Open* 2, no. 1 (February 2012): e000435. doi:10.1136/bmjopen-2011-000435.

Bielinski, S. J., J. E. Olson, J. Pathak, R. M. Weinshilboum, L. Wang, K. J. Lyke, E. Ryu, et al. "Preemptive Genotyping for Personalized Medicine: Design of the Right Drug, Right Dose, Right Time—Using Genomic Data to Individualize Treatment Protocol." *Mayo Clinic Proceedings* 89, no. 1 (January 2014): 25–33. doi:10.1016/j.mayocp.2013.10.021. PubMed (PMID: 24388019). PubMed Central (PMC3932754).

Block, Andrew R., Ephrem Fernandez, and Edwin Kremer, eds. *Handbook of Pain Syndromes: Biopsychosocial Perspectives*. New York: Psychology Press, 2013.

Boivin, A., K. Currie, B. Fervers, J. Gracia, M. James, C. Marshall, et al. "Patient and Public Involvement in Clinical Guidelines: International Experiences and Future Perspectives." *Quality and Safety Health Care* 19, no. 5 (October 2010): e22. doi:10.1136/qshc.2009.034835. PubMed (PMID: 20427302).

Bookstein, L., S. S. Gidding, M. Donovan, and F. A. Smith. "Day-to-Day Variability of Serum Cholesterol, Triglyceride, and High-Density Lipoprotein Cholesterol Levels." *Archives of Internal Medicine* 150, no. 8 (August 1990): 1653–57. doi:10.1001/archinte.1990.00040031653012.

Borden, W. B., Y. P. Chiang, and R. Kronick. "Bringing Patient-Centered Outcomes Research to Life" (review). *Value Health* 18, no. 4 (June 2015): 355–57. doi:10.1016/j.jval.2015.01.010. PubMed (PMID: 26091588).

Borgerson, Kirstin. "Valuing Evidence: Bias and the Evidence Hierarchy of Evidence-Based Medicine." *Perspectives in Biology and Medicine* 52, no. 2 (2009): 218–33.

Bowlby, John. *Loss: Sadness and Depression*. Attachment and Loss 3. New York: Basic Books, 1980.

Buckius, Michelle T., Brian McGrath, John Monk, Rod Grim, Theodore Bell, and Vanita Ahuja. "Changing Epidemiology of Acute Appendicitis in the United States: Study Period 1993–2008." *Journal of Surgical Research* 175, no. 2 (2012): 185–90.

Bylander, Jessica. "Civil Unrest, Police Use of Force, and the Public's Health." *Health Affairs* 34, no. 8 (2015): 1264–68.

Cappola, Anne R., and Susan J. Mandel. "Improving the Long-Term Management of Benign Thyroid Nodules." *Journal of the American Medical Association* 313, no. 9 (2015): 903–4.

Centers for Disease Control and Prevention. *Wide-Ranging Online Data for Epidemiologic Research (WONDER)*. Last reviewed September 17, 2015. http://wonder.cdc.gov/mortsql.html.

Chien, A. T., and M. B. Rosenthal. "Waste Not, Want Not: Promoting Efficient Use of Health Care Resources." *Annals of Internal Medicine* 158 (2013): 67–68. doi:10.7326/0003-4819-158-1-201301010-00014.

Childs, B., C. Weiner, and D. Valle. "A Science of the Individual: Implications for a Medical School Curriculum." *Annual Review of Genomics and Human Genetics* 6 (2005): 313–30.

Concato, J., N. Shah, and R. I. Horwitz. "Randomized, Controlled Trials, Observational Studies, and the Hierarchy of Research Designs." *New England Journal of Medicine* 342, no. 25 (June 2000): 1887–92. PubMed (PMID: 10861325). PubMed Central (PMC1557642).

Cuffee, Yendelela, Chinwe Ogedegbe, Natasha J. Williams, Gbenga Ogedegbe, and Antoinette Schoenthaler. "Psychosocial Risk Factors for Hypertension: An Update of the Literature" (review). *Current Hypertension Reports* 16, no. 10 (October 2014): 1–11. doi:10.1007/s11906-014-0483-3. PubMed (PMID: 25139781). PubMed Central (PMC4163921).

Davis, Karen, Kristof Stremikis, David Squires, and Cathy Schoen. *Mirror, Mirror on the Wall: How the Performance of the U.S. Health Care System Compares Internationally: 2014 Update*. New York: Commonwealth Fund, 2014. Accessed September 21, 2015. www.commonwealthfund.org/~/media/files/publications/fund-report/2014/jun/1755_davis_mirror_mirror_2014.pdf.

Dean, B. B., A. D. Gano Jr., K. Knight, J. J. Ofman, and R. Fass. "Effectiveness of Proton Pump Inhibitors in Nonerosive Reflux Disease" (review). *Clinical Gastroenterology and Hepatology* 2, no. 8 (August 2004): 656–64. PubMed (PMID: 15290657).

Denk, F., S. B. McMahon, and I. Tracey. "Pain Vulnerability: A Neurobiological Perspective." *Nature Neuroscience* 17, no. 2 (February 2014): 192–200.

Dimidjian, S., S. D. Hollon, K. S. Dobson, K. B. Schmaling, R. J. Kohlenberg, M. E. Addis, R. Gallop, et al. "Randomized Trial of Behavioral Activation, Cognitive Therapy, and Antidepressant Medication in the Acute Treatment of Adults with Major Depression." *Journal of Consulting and Clinical Psychology* 74, no. 4 (August 2006): 658–70. doi:10.1037/0022-006X.74.4.658.

Donner, Allan. "A Bayesian Approach to the Interpretation of Subgroup Results in Clinical Trials." *Journal of Chronic Diseases* 35, no. 6 (1982): 429–35.

Donner-Banzhoff, N., and A. Sönnichsen. "Strategies for Prescribing Statins." *British Medical Journal* 336, no. 7639 (February 2008): 288–89. doi:10.1136/bmj.39387.573947.80. PubMed (PMID: 18258935). PubMed Central (PMC2234555).

Doyle, Joseph J., John A. Graves, Jonathan Gruber, and Samuel A. Kleiner. "Measuring Returns to Hospital Care: Evidence from Ambulance Referral Patterns." *Journal of Political Economy* 123, no. 1 (2015): 170–214.

Eccleston, C., A. C. Williams, and W. S. Rogers. "Patients' and Professionals' Understandings of the Causes of Chronic Pain: Blame, Responsibility and Identity Protection." *Social Science and Medicine* 45, no. 5 (September 1997): 699–709.

Edelson, J. T., M. C. Weinstein, A. N. Tosteson, L. Williams, T. H. Lee, and L. Goldman. "Long-Term Cost-Effectiveness of Various Initial Monotherapies for Mild to Moderate Hypertension." *Journal of the American Medical Association* 263, no. 3 (1990): 407–13. doi:10.1001/jama.1990.03440030094028.

Edwards, Adrian, and Glyn Elwyn. *Shared Decision-Making in Health Care: Achieving Evidence-Based Patient Choice*. Oxford: Oxford University Press, 2009.

Egan, Brent M., Yumin Zhao, and R. Neal Axon. "US Trends in Prevalence, Awareness, Treatment, and Control of Hypertension, 1988–2008." *Journal of the American Medical Association* 303, no. 20 (May 2010): 2043–50. doi:10.1001/jama.2010.650.

Ellenberg, Jordan. *How Not to Be Wrong: The Power of Mathematical Thinking*. New York: Penguin, 2014.

Emanuel, Ezekiel J., and Linda L. Emanuel. "Four Models of the Physician-Patient Relationship." *Journal of the American Medical Association* 267, no. 16 (1992): 2221–26.

Engel, G. L. "The Need for a New Medical Model: A Challenge for Biomedicine." *Science* 196, no. 4286 (April 1977): 129–36. doi:10.1126/science.847460.

Etzion, O., and M. G. Ghany. "A Cure for the High Cost of Hepatitis C Virus Treatment." *Annals of Internal Medicine* 162 (2015): 660–61. doi:10.7326/M15-0674.

Farmer, M. E., B. Z. Locke, E. K. Mościcki, A. L. Dannenberg, D. B. Larson, and L. S. Radloff. "Physical Activity and Depressive Symptoms: The NHANES I Epidemiologic Follow-Up Study." *American Journal of Epidemiology* 128, no. 6 (December 1988): 1340–51. PubMed (PMID: 3264110).

Fields, H. L. "The Doctor's Dilemma: Opiate Analgesics and Chronic Pain." *Neuron* 69, no. 4 (February 2011): 591–94. doi:10.1016/j.neuron.2011.02.001. PubMed (PMID: 21338871). PubMed Central (PMC3073133).

Flum, David R. "Acute Appendicitis—Appendectomy or the 'Antibiotics First' Strategy." *New England Journal of Medicine* 372, no. 20 (2015): 1937–43.

Foreman, Judy. *A Nation in Pain: Healing Our Biggest Health Problem*. Oxford: Oxford University Press, 2014.

Furlan, A. D., J. A. Sandoval, A. Mailis-Gagnon, and E. Tunks. "Opioids for Chronic Noncancer Pain: A Meta-analysis of Effectiveness and Side Effects." *Canadian Medical Association Journal* 174, no. 11 (May 2006): 1589–94. PubMed (PMID: 16717269). PubMed Central (PMC1459894).

Giugliano, Dario, Maria Ida Maiorino, Giuseppe Bellastella, Michela Petrizzo, Antonio Ceriello, Stefano Genovese, and Katherine Esposito. "Setting the Hemoglobin A1C Target in Type 2 Diabetes: A Priori, A Posteriori, or Neither?" *Endocrine* 50, no. 1 (2015): 56–60.

Grady, Deborah, and Rita F. Redberg. "Less Is More: How Less Health Care Can Result in Better Health." *Archives of Internal Medicine* 170, no. 9 (2010): 749–50.

Graham, D. Y., Y.-C. Lee, M.-S. Wu. "Rational *Helicobacter pylori* Therapy: Evidence-Based Medicine Rather Than Medicine-Based Evidence." *Clinical Gastroenterology and Hepatol-*

ogy 12, no. 2 (February 2014): 177–86.e3; Discussion e12–e13. doi:10.1016/j.cgh.2013.05.028. PubMed (PMID: 23751282). PubMed Central (PMC3830667).

Graham, D. Y., G. M. Lew, P. D. Klein, D. G. Evans, D. J. Evans Jr., Z. A. Saeed, and H. M. Malaty. "Effect of Treatment of *Helicobacter pylori* Infection on the Long-Term Recurrence of Gastric or Duodenal Ulcer: A Randomized, Controlled Study." *Annals of Internal Medicine* 116, no. 9 (1992): 705–8. doi:10.7326/0003-4819-116-9-705.

Gui, G. P., C. V. Cheruvu, N. West, K. Sivaniah, and A. G. Fiennes. "Is Cholecystectomy Effective Treatment for Symptomatic Gallstones? Clinical Outcome after Long-Term Follow-Up" (review). *Annals of the Royal College of Surgeons of England* 80, no. 1 (January 1998): 25–32. PubMed (PMID: 9579123). PubMed Central (PMC2502763).

Guo, Fangjian, Di He, Wei Zhang, and R. Grace Walton. "Trends in Prevalence, Awareness, Management, and Control of Hypertension among United States Adults, 1999 to 2010." *Journal of the American College of Cardiology* 60, no. 7 (2012): 599–606. doi:10.1016/j.jacc.2012.04.026.

Hellemons, M. E., J. Kerschbaum, S. Bakker, H. Neuwirt, B. Mayer, G. Mayer, D. de Zeeuw, H. J. Lambers Heerspink, and M. Rudnicki. "Validity of Biomarkers Predicting Onset or Progression of Nephropathy in Patients with Type 2 Diabetes: A Systematic Review." *Diabetic Medicine* 29 (2012): 567–77. doi:10.1111/j.1464-5491.2011.03437.x.

Hussey, P. S., S. Wertheimer, and A. Mehrotra. "The Association between Health Care Quality and Cost: A Systematic Review." *Annals of Internal Medicine* 158 (2013): 27–34. doi:10.7326/0003-4819-158-1-201301010-00006.

Inzucchi, S., and S. Majumdar. "Glycemic Targets: What Is the Evidence?" (review). *Medical Clinics of North America* 99, no. 1 (January 2015): 47–67. doi:10.1016/j.mcna.2014.08.018. Erratum: *Medical Clinics of North America* 99, no. 2 (March 2015): xix.

Ioannidis, John P. A. "Why Most Published Research Findings Are False." *Chance* 18, no. 4 (2005): 40–47.

Jager, Leah R., and Jeffrey T. Leek. "An Estimate of the Science-Wise False Discovery Rate and Application to the Top Medical Literature." *Biostatistics* 15, no. 1 (2014): 1–12.

Joynt, K. E., E. J. Orav, and A. K. Jha. "The Association between Hospital Volume and Processes, Outcomes, and Costs of Care for Congestive Heart Failure." *Annals of Internal Medicine* 154 (2011): 94–102. doi:10.7326/0003-4819-154-2-201101180-00008.

Kaplan, Sherrie H., Barbara Gandek, Sheldon Greenfield, William H. Rogers, and John E. Ware Jr. "Patient and Visit Characteristics Related to Physicians' Participatory Decision-Making Style: Results from the Medical Outcomes Study." *Medical Care* 33, no. 12 (December 1995): 1176–87. www.jstor.org/stable/3766817.

Kayton, Wayne, Ming-Yu Fan, Jürgen Unützer, Jennifer Taylor, Harold Pincus, and Michael Schoenbaum. "Depression and Diabetes: A Potentially Lethal Combination." *Journal of General Internal Medicine* 23, no. 10 (2008): 1571–75.

Khan, Khalid, Regina Kunz, Jos Kleijnen, and Gerd Antes. *Systematic Reviews to Support Evidence-Based Medicine*. 2nd ed. Boca Raton, FL, and London: CRC Press, 2011.

Khoury, M. J., and J. P. Evans. "A Public Health Perspective on a National Precision Medicine Cohort: Balancing Long-Term Knowledge Generation with Early Health Benefit." *Journal of the American Medical Association* 313, no. 21 (2015): 2117–18. doi:10.1001/jama.2015.3382.

Korenstein, D., R. Falk, E. A. Howell, T. Bishop, and S. Keyhani. "Overuse of Health Care Services in the United States: An Understudied Problem." *Archives of Internal Medicine* 172, no. 2 (2012): 171–78. doi:10.1001/archinternmed.2011.772.

Lichtenberg, Frank R. "The Effects of Medicare on Health Care Utilization and Outcomes." *Forum for Health Economics and Policy* 5, no. 1 (January 2002). doi:10.2202/1558-9544.1028.

Lipska, K. J., J. S. Ross, Y. Miao, N. D. Shah, S. J. Lee, and M. A. Steinman. "Potential Overtreatment of Diabetes Mellitus in Older Adults with Tight Glycemic Control." *JAMA Internal Medicine* 175, no. 3 (2015): 356–62.

Lumley, Thomas. "Network Meta-analysis for Indirect Treatment Comparisons." *Statistics in Medicine* 21, no. 16 (2002): 2313–24.

MacDorman, Marian F., Fay Menacker, and Eugene Declercq. "Cesarean Birth in the United States: Epidemiology, Trends, and Outcomes." *Clinics in Perinatology* 35, no. 2 (2008): 293–307.

Manderson, Lenore, and Carolyn Smith-Morris. *Chronic Conditions, Fluid States: Chronicity and the Anthropology of Illness.* New Brunswick, NJ: Rutgers University Press, 2010.

Martin, S. S., and R. S. Blumenthal. "Concepts and Controversies: The 2013 American College of Cardiology/American Heart Association Risk Assessment and Cholesterol Treatment Guidelines." *Annals of Internal Medicine* 160 (2014): 356–58. doi:10.7326/M13-2805.

McNicol, E. D., A. Midbari, and E. Eisenberg. "Opioids for Neuropathic Pain." *Cochrane Database of Systematic Reviews*, no. 8 (2013). Article no. CD006146. doi:10.1002/14651858.CD006146.pub2.

Methodology Committee of the Patient-Centered Outcomes Research Institute (PCORI). "Methodological Standards and Patient-Centeredness in Comparative Effectiveness Research: The PCORI Perspective." *Journal of the American Medical Association* 307, no. 15 (2012): 1636–40.

Moll, Annemarie. *The Logic of Care: Health and the Problem of Patient Choice.* London and New York: Routledge, 2008.

Morley, S., C. Eccleston, and A. Williams. "Systematic Review and Meta-analysis of Randomized Controlled Trials of Cognitive Behaviour Therapy and Behaviour Therapy for Chronic Pain in Adults, Excluding Headache." *PAIN* 80, no. 1–2 (March 1999): 1–13. PubMed (PMID: 10204712).

Moyer, V. A., and the U.S. Preventive Services Task Force. "Vitamin, Mineral, and Multivitamin Supplements for the Primary Prevention of Cardiovascular Disease and Cancer: U.S. Preventive Services Task Force Recommendation Statement." *Annals of Internal Medicine* 160 (2014): 558–64. doi:10.7326/M14-0198.

National Institute of Diabetes and Digestive and Kidney Diseases. *The A1C Test and Diabetes.* NIH Publication 14-7816 (March 2014). www.niddk.nih.gov/health-information/health-topics/diagnostic-tests/a1c-test-diabetes/Pages/index.aspx#15.

Nelson, Lewis S., David N. Juurlink, and Jeanmarie Perrone. "Addressing the Opioid Epidemic." *Journal of the American Medical Association* 314, no. 14 (2015): 1453–54.

O'Connor, E. A., E. P. Whitlock, T. L. Beil, and B. N. Gaynes. "Screening for Depression in Adult Patients in Primary Care Settings: A Systematic Evidence Review." *Annals of Internal Medicine* 151 (2009): 793–803. doi:10.7326/0003-4819-151-11-200912010-0.

Ojala, T., A. Häkkinen, J. Karppinen, K. Sipilä, T. Suutama, and A. Piirainen. "The Dominance of Chronic Pain: A Phenomenological Study." *Musculoskeletal Care*, January 15, 2014. doi:10.1002/msc.1066.

Okie, Susan. "A Flood of Opiates, a Rising Tide of Deaths." *New England Journal of Medicine* 363 (2010): 1981–85. doi:10.1056/NEJMp1011512.

Paul, Laurie Ann. *Transformative Experience.* Oxford: Oxford University Press, 2014.

Piper, M. A., C. V. Evans, B. U. Burda, E. O'Connor, E. P. Whitlock, and K. L. Margolis. "Diagnostic and Predictive Accuracy of Blood Pressure Screening Methods with Consideration of Rescreening Intervals: A Systematic Review for the U.S. Preventive Services Task Force." *Annals of Internal Medicine* 162 (2015): 192–204. doi:10.7326/M14-1539.

Polanyi, Michael, and Amartya Sen. *The Tacit Dimension.* New York: Doubleday, 1967.

Rand, L. I., and F. L. Ferris III. "Long-Term Contributions from the Diabetes Control and Complications Trial Cohort." *JAMA Ophthalmology*, August 13, 2015. doi:10.1001/jamaophthalmol.2015.2735.

Rao, Vijay M., and David C. Levin. "The Overuse of Diagnostic Imaging and the Choosing Wisely Initiative." *Annals of Internal Medicine* 157, no. 8 (2012): 574–76.

Reames, Bradley N., Amir A. Ghaferi, John D. Birkmeyer, and Justin B. Dimick. "Hospital Volume and Operative Mortality in the Modern Era." *Annals of Surgery* 260, no. 2 (August 2014): 244–51. doi:10.1097/SLA.0000000000000375.

Redelmeier, Donald A., and Eldar Shafir. "Medical Decision Making in Situations That Offer Multiple Alternatives." *Journal of the American Medical Association* 273, no. 4 (1995): 302–5.

Ridker, P. M., and N. R. Cook. "Comparing Cardiovascular Risk Prediction Scores." *Annals of Internal Medicine* 162 (2015): 313–14. doi:10.7326/M14-2820.

Roberts, Marc J., and Michael R. Reich. "Ethical Analysis in Public Health." *Lancet* 359, no. 9311 (2002): 1055–59.

Roddy, E., W. Zhang, and M. Doherty. "Aerobic Walking or Strengthening Exercise for Osteoarthritis of the Knee? A Systematic Review." *Annals Rheumatic Diseases* 64, no. 4 (April 2005): 544–48. PubMed (PMID: 15769914). PubMed Central (PMC1755453).

Rost, Kathryn, Paul Nutting, Jeffrey Smith, James Werner, and Naihua Duan. "Improving Depression Outcomes in Community Primary Care Practice." *Journal of General Internal Medicine* 16, no. 3 (2001): 143–49.

Rubin, R. "Precision Medicine: The Future or Simply Politics?" *Journal of the American Medical Association* 313, no. 11 (2015): 1089–91. doi:10.1001/jama.2015.0957.

Samuelson, William, and Richard Zeckhauser. "Status Quo Bias in Decision Making." *Journal of Risk and Uncertainty* 1, no. 1 (1988): 7–59.

Silva-Néto, R. P., K. J. Almeida, and S. N. Bernardino. "Analysis of the Duration of Migraine Prophylaxis." *Journal of the Neurological Sciences* 337, no. 1–2 (February 2014): 38–41. doi:10.1016/j.jns.2013.11.013. PubMed (PMID: 24308946).

Silver, Nate. *The Signal and the Noise: Why So Many Predictions Fail—but Some Don't.* New York: Penguin, 2012.

SPRINT Research Group. "A Randomized Trial of Intensive versus Standard Blood-Pressure Control. *New England Journal of Medicine* 373, no. 22 (November 2015): 2103–16. doi:10.1056/NEJMoa1511939. PubMed (PMID: 26551272).

Srinivas, S. V., R. A. Deyo, and Z. D. Berger. "Application of 'Less Is More' to Low Back Pain." *Archives of Internal Medicine* 172, no. 13 (July 2012): 1016–20. doi:10.1001/archinternmed.2012.1838.

Stefan, Norbert, Hans-Ulrich Häring, Frank B. Hu, and Matthias B. Schulze. "Metabolically Healthy Obesity: Epidemiology, Mechanisms, and Clinical Implications." *Lancet: Diabetes and Endocrinology* 1, no. 2 (2013): 152–62.

Stiggelbout, A. M., A. H. Pieterse, and J. C. De Haes. "Shared Decision Making: Concepts, Evidence, and Practice." *Patient Education and Counseling* 90, no. 10 (October 2015): 1172–79. doi:10.1016/j.pec.2015.06.022. PubMed (PMID: 26215573).

Stone, Neil J., Jennifer G. Robinson, Alice H. Lichtenstein, C. Noel Bairey Merz, Conrad B. Blum, Robert H. Eckel, Anne C. Goldberg, et al. "2013 ACC/AHA Guideline on the Treatment of Blood Cholesterol to Reduce Atherosclerotic Cardiovascular Risk in Adults." *Journal of the American College of Cardiologists* 63, no. 25_PA (July 2014): 2889–934. doi:10.1016/j.jacc.2013.11.002.

Sydenham, Thomas. *The Works of Thomas Sydenham, MD, on Acute and Chronic Diseases: With Their Histories and Modes of Cure.* Philadelphia: B. & T. Kite, 1809. Research Publications Early American Medical Imprints collection reel 91, no. 1845.

Timmermans, Stefan, and Emily S. Kolker. "Evidence-Based Medicine and the Reconfiguration of Medical Knowledge." In "Health and Health Care in the United States: Origins and Dynamics," extra issue, *Journal of Health and Social Behavior* 45 (2004): 177–93.

Tversky, Amos, and Daniel Kahneman. "The Framing of Decisions and the Psychology of Choice." *Science* 211, no. 4481 (1981): 453–58.

Ubel, Peter. *Critical Decisions: How You and Your Doctor Can Make the Right Medical Choices Together.* New York: HarperCollins, 2012.

Van Spall, H. C., A. Toren, A. Kiss, and R. A. Fowler. "Eligibility Criteria of Randomized Controlled Trials Published in High-Impact General Medical Journals: A Systematic Sampling Review." *Journal of the American Medical Association* 297, no. 11 (2007): 1233–40. doi:10.1001/jama.297.11.1233.

Verghese, Abraham, and Ralph I. Horwitz. "In Praise of the Physical Examination." *British Medical Journal* 339 (2009): b5448. doi:10.1136/bmj.b5448.

Vergunst, F. K., A. Fekadu, S. C. Wooderson, C. S. Tunnard, L. J. Rane, K. Markopoulou, and A. J. Cleare. "Longitudinal Course of Symptom Severity and Fluctuation in Patients with Treatment-Resistant Unipolar and Bipolar Depression." *Psychiatry Research* 207, no. 3 (May 2013): 143–49. doi:10.1016/j.psychres.2013.03.022. PubMed (PMID: 23601791).

Von Korff, Michael, Andrew Kolodny, Richard A. Deyo, and Roger Chou. "Long-Term Opi-oid Therapy Reconsidered." *Annals of Internal Medicine* 155, no. 5 (September 2011): 325–28.

Walraven, C. van, and C. D. Naylor. "Do We Know What Inappropriate Laboratory Utilization Is? A Systematic Review of Laboratory Clinical Audits." *Journal of the American Medical Association* 280 (1998): 550–58.

Weber, M. A., E. L. Schiffrin, W. B. White, S. Mann, L. H. Lindholm, J. G. Kenerson, J. M. Flack, et al. "Clinical Practice Guidelines for the Management of Hypertension in the Community: A Statement by the American Society of Hypertension and the International Society of Hypertension." *Journal of Clinical Hypertension* 16, no. 1 (January 2014): 14–26. doi:10.1111/jch.12237. PubMed (PMID: 24341872).

Whelton, P. K. "The Elusiveness of Population-Wide High Blood Pressure Control." *Annual Review of Public Health* 36 (March 18, 2015): 109–30. doi:10.1146/annurev-publhealth-031914-122949. PubMed (PMID: 25594330).

Wijeysundera, H. C., and D. T. Ko. "Does Percutaneous Coronary Intervention Reduce Mortal-ity in Patients with Stable Chronic Angina: Are We Talking about Apples and Oranges?" *Circulation: Cardiovascular Quality Outcomes* 2, no. 2 (March 2009): 123–26. doi:10.1161/CIRCOUTCOMES.108.834853. PubMed (PMID: 20031824).

Wilkinson, Richard G., and Michael Gideon Marmot. *Social Determinants of Health: The Solid Facts*. 2nd ed. Copenhagen: World Health Organization, Regional Office for Europe, 2003.

Wolpe, Paul Root. "The Triumph of Autonomy in American Bioethics: A Sociological View." In *Bioethics and Society: Constructing the Ethical Enterprise*, edited by Raymond G. De Vries and Janardan Subedi, 38–59. Upper Saddle River, NJ: Prentice Hall, 1998.

Wright, J. T. "The Benefits of Detecting and Treating Mild Hypertension: What We Know, and What We Need to Learn." *Annals of Internal Medicine* 162 (2015): 233–34. doi:10.7326/M14-2836.

INDEX

Affordable Care Act, 1, 28, 35, 36, 42, 48
American College of Cardiology (ACC), 107, 108
American Diabetes Association, 76, 78
American Heart Association (AHA), 107, 108
aneurysm, 133–134
angina, treatment of, 120–121
Annals of Internal Medicine, 34, 116
Aristotle, 56
arthritis, 83–92, 97; ameliorative treatment of, 92; biomedical treatment of, 84–85; and decision making, 86–87, 88–89, 91–92; and diabetes, 86–87; and doctor-patient relationships, 90–91; and surgery, 85–86, 87–88
atrial fibrillation, 1–3

Baltimore, 1, 46, 95, 131
Beswick, Andrew David, 87
biomedical paradigm, 32, 72, 131, 132, 137–148; shortcomings of, 73–74, 139–141
blood pressure: treatment of, 2, 12–13, 38, 146–147. *See also* hypertension
BMJ Open, 87
British Medical Journal, 72, 139. *See also* Smith, Robert

cardiac risk calculator, 110, 111, 112
Charon, Rita, 30

chronic conditions, 24–26. *See also* chronic pain; depression
chronic pain, 11–21; definition and diagnosis of, 15–16; management of, 13. *See also* opioids
Coates, Ta-Nehisi, 41
colon cancer, screening for, 36–37
CT scan, 133, 134. *See also* aneurysm
cure: absence of, 25–26; and arthritis, 92; and diabetes, 80–81; uncertainty of, 26–27

Dartmouth Health Care Atlas, 42
decision making, 2–7, 72, 74–75; and arthritis, 86–87, 88–89, 91–92; and depression, 51–56; and diabetes, 72–74; guidelines for, 7–9; and hypertension, 61–62, 63–64; and individual needs, 34, 138; and medical guidelines, 104; and surgery, 93–95, 97–100
depression, 28, 45–58; control of, 46–47; and diabetes, 5, 6; and doctor-patient relationships, 46, 48–51; and health services, 54–55; and high blood pressure, 62–64; and self-care, 55–58; treatment of, 47–48, 51–52, 84–85
diabetes, 71–81, 127–128; and precision medicine, 79–81; self-treatment of, 76–77
diagnosis, 15–16, 26–27, 127–128, 145; and advice seeking, 72–76; and

personhood, 140; and prestige, 142; and
public health, 140. *See also* decision
making
*Diagnostic and Statistical Manual of
Mental Disorders* (*DSM-5*), 47
doctor-patient relationships, 1–3, 4–5,
13–14, 19–21, 90–92, 127–128. *See
also* shared decision making

Elias, Peter, 107
Engel, George. *See* psychosocial medicine
evidence-based medicine, 4, 17–21, 72,
107, 137–138
evidence-informed medicine, 107

false certainty, 127–135; and health care,
129–130; and health disparities, 131;
patient strategies, 130, 131–132; and
treatment options, 132. *See also* health
Framingham study, 78, 110. *See also*
diabetes; heart disease

"Guideline on the Treatment of Blood
Cholesterol to Reduce Atherosclerotic
Cardiovascular Risk in Adults," 107,
108, 109–110, 111. *See also* American
College of Cardiology; American Heart
Association
guidelines. *See* medical guidelines

health, 139; common sense and, 144–145;
social determinants of, 64–65,
143–144; spectrum of conditions for,
139. *See also* wellness
health care data: online, 95–96, 124–125;
qualitative versus quantitative, 124
health care system: and African
Americans, 41; and cost, 41–43; and
economic access, 34, 36–37, 41–44;
and inequality, 7–8, 39, 44, 141
Health Expectations, 87
HealthGrades.com, 96
heart disease, 40, 78, 84, 109. *See also*
blood pressure; Framingham study
hypertension, 59–69; and anxiety, 62–63,
64, 65, 66; medication, 62, 63, 67–69;
monitoring of, 65–66; treatment of,
59–61, 66–69

individualistic care, 31–32. *See also*
science of the individual
individualized medicine, 31

Jager, Leah, 118–119
*Journal of the American Medical
Association*, 147

Kahneman, Daniel, 94

Leek, Jeffrey, 118–119
Lehman, Richard, 72–73
The Logic of Care. See Moll, Annemarie

Medicaid, 34
medical guidelines, 103–113; conflicts of
interest in, 106; interpretation of,
110–113; making of, 103–104,
105–113; practical application of,
104–105
medical research, 115–125. *See also*
patient-centered care
medical science, 8–9, 106, 115–117,
121–122
Medicare, 35
migraine, 141–142
Moll, Annemarie, 46, 72, 74, 130

narrative medicine: collective, 29–30;
individual, 30
National Institutes of Health, 28, 147
network meta-analysis, 121. *See also*
statistics

Obama, Barack, 99, 147
ObamaCare, 28, 34
opioids, 13–14, 16–17
orthopedics, 95, 97, 98

pain, 14, 83–84. *See also* chronic pain
patient autonomy, 37, 88–89, 138
patient-centered care, 17–21, 28–29,
123–125
Patient-Centered Outcomes Research
Institute (PCORI), 28, 74, 117
patient-related outcomes, 40
Paul, L. A., 135
personal care, 5–9; guidelines for, 7–9
phronesis, 56, 72, 122